RADIOGRAPHIC ASSESSMENT *for* NURSES

RADIOGRAPHIC ASSESSMENT *for* NURSES

Patricia A. Dettenmeier, RN, MSN(R), CCRN
Pulmonary Clinical Nurse Specialist
Assistant Clinical Professor of Nursing
Instructor in Medicine
St. Louis University Health Sciences Center
St. Louis, Missouri

with 150 illustrations

Mosby

St. Louis Baltimore Berlin Boston Carlsbad Chicago London Madrid
Naples New York Philadelphia Sydney Tokyo Toronto

Mosby
Dedicated to Publishing Excellence

Editor: Timothy M. Griswold
Developmental Editor: Jolynn Gower
Project Manager: Gayle May Morris
Production Editor: Lisa Marcus
Manufacturing Supervisor: Betty Richmond
Design Manager: Susan Lane
Cover Design: GW Graphics

Printed in the United States of America
Composition by Top Graphics
Printing/binding by Maple-Vail Book Mfg. Group

Mosby–Year Book, Inc.
11830 Westline Industrial Drive
St. Louis, Missouri 63146

International Standard Book Number 0-8016-7245-7

97 98 / 9 8 7 6 5 4

Contributor

Connie A. Walleck, RN, MS, FCCM
Director, Critical Care and Emergency Nursing
University Hospital
Syracuse, New York

Acknowledgments

Thanks to all the physicians, nurses, radiation technologists, and staff at St. Louis University Health Sciences Center who helped locate the radiographs for this text.

Patricia A. Dettenmeier

Contents

1 Radiographic Assessment for Nurses

X-ray films have revolutionized the diagnosis and treatment of patients, especially in the past two decades with the development of newer technologies. The plain x-ray film (or more formally radiograph) was first developed in the late 1800s by Professor Wilhelm Conrad Roentgen. This simple technique is now accompanied by fluoroscopy, nuclear medicine scintigraphy (such as ventilation-perfusion, gallium, or indium scans), angiography (such as venograms, and pulmonary or cerebral angiograms), computerized axial tomography (CAT or CT scan), magnetic resonance imaging (MRI), and positive electron transmission (PET scan). High doses of radiation therapy administered to a circumscribed area are used for reducing tumor bulk, decreasing pain from bone metastases, or obliterating cancer cells.

X-ray films were formerly performed, interpreted, and stored only in the radiology department. Physicians spoke directly with the radiologist for interpretation or awaited posting of the reports in the patient's chart. These procedures caused some delays in the treatment of the patient. Currently, portable x-ray machines and nuclear medicine scanners can be taken to the patient's room when the patient is unable to go to the radiology department, and interpretation of the film occurs in or near the patient's room. In many hospitals and health care centers, viewing boxes are available in the physicians' office and patient care areas. Some intensive care units have elaborate viewing areas or rooms that allow serial x-rays to be stored or viewed.

The ability to examine x-ray films in or near the patient's room has undoubtedly enhanced patient care, especially in the intensive care unit. Caregivers can quickly assess placement of catheters, tubes, and prostheses, determine presence and estimate volume of fluids or air in interior body cavities such as the head and chest, identify disease processes such as organomegaly or airway obstruction, and judge the extent and type of bone injuries. Serial films also are useful in determining the effects of therapy such as diuretics, chest tubes, skeletal traction, antibiotics, and chest therapy.

Interpretation and report of the findings is the responsibility of the resident or attending physician. In most cases the radiologist officially interprets and reports the findings on a film, although other physicians may examine the film and note findings in their progress notes. The goal of this book is to prepare the nurse to assess an x-ray film for gross abnormalities that may influence patient care. The nurse has the responsibility to report findings to the physician for confirmation and intervention.

PRINCIPLES OF RADIOLOGY

X-ray Beams

X-ray beams were accidentally discovered by Wilhelm Conrad Roentgen in 1895. Despite what was learned about the diagnostic and adverse effects of x-ray beams in the next 15 years, radiation safety procedures were not instituted until the 1930s. High doses of radiation can cause cutaneous dermatitis, atrophy (shrinking) of tissues, dysfunction (improper metabolism), hematologic depression, gonadal sterility, cataracts (if directed at the lens of the eye), and malignant diseases, especially leukemia (Ballinger, 1991). Since x-ray examinations are commonly performed outside the radiology department, especially in critical care and emergency areas, it is important for nurses to understand the principles of wave travel and the appropriate safety precautions.

Principles of Wave Travel. Energizing an x-ray tube results in the emission of collimated x-ray beams. This is analogous to the light emitted from a flashlight. As the beam travels through the air, ionization occurs and energy is deposited in the air. This deposition of energy is called exposure, and the unit by which it is measured is the roentgen (R). An exposure of 1 R produces 2.08×10^9 ionizations in a cubic centimeter of air at standard temperature and pressure. When the energy meets an object, ionization is deposited and referred to as radiation exposure. The dose of absorbed radiation is measured in rads. One rad is equivalent to depositing 100 ergs of energy in 1 gram (g) of the irradiated object. In the hospital and other health care facilities, the radiation dose resulting from occupational exposure is measured in radiation dose equivalent or radiation equivalent man (rem). One rem is equivalent to 100 ergs/g. The difference between rad and rem is that rem refers to occupational exposure and is usually the result of scatter. In diagnostic radiology, unlike the nuclear power or research industries, 1 R is considered equal to 1 rad and to 1 rem. In the hospital setting, radiation exposure is generally 1000 times less and is referred to as milliroentgen (mR), millirad (mrad), or millirem (mrem).

Annual radiation exposure of a healthy individual is about 200 mrad/yr. (Note: radiologic technologists receive approximately another 100 mrad/yr, mostly from fluoroscopy and portable radiography. The exposure to most critical care and emergency nurses who wear protective apparel, especially during fluoroscopic procedures such as pulmonary artery catheter insertion, should be considerably less.) This exposure comes from many sources. Among these sources are background radiation sources. Background radiation sources include naturally occurring radionucleotides in the earth like uranium or cosmic radiation from the sun, or internal radionucleotides naturally deposited in the body like potassium 40. People receive various levels of radiation from medical, diagnostic, and therapeutic interventions, from industrial exposure, and from research applications of ionizing radiation. Recent reports of radiation from video display terminals, television receivers, and airport security (detection) devices have received much attention with regard to exposure and infertility (Ballinger, 1991).

The central x-ray beam is perpendicular to the patient's body in most instances. The focus of the beam is limited to irradiate only the area under examination. This focus reduces scatter radiation and secondary irradiation of surrounding structures or individuals. This restriction of the beam is accomplished by the use of metallic or lead shutters, diaphragms, or collimators, which absorb the radiation.

Direction of Wave. Although many radiographs must be taken in the radiology department because of the equipment required, some standard views can be taken in the patient's room with portable radiographic equipment. Radiographs taken in the radiology department are generally of better quality because the environment and procedures in the radiology department are more controlled and standardized and the equipment is better. Because the quality of the radiograph affects the ability of the radiologist to identify patient abnormalities, it is important to try to obtain all radiographs under the best conditions. Patients who can be safely transported to the radiology department for the radiograph should do so to obtain the best quality film.

Radiographs are taken with patients in a variety of positions. Positioning depends on the type of imaging procedure, the inner structures to be viewed, the age and condition of the patient, and the technologist performing the procedure. Examination of the head, including the sinuses, is usually performed with the patient recumbent or sitting, although the standing position is used in some types of head radiographs. Neck and spine radiographs are usually performed with the patient in a recumbent position. Chest radiographs are ideally performed with the patient standing, especially in the outpatient setting, although a sitting position may also be used. With acutely ill patients a sitting or recumbent position is often necessary. Abdominal radiographs are usually taken with the patient in a recumbent or upright position.

X-ray beams are directed to penetrate the body from posterior, anterior, or lateral positions. In the following discussions, chest radiograph positions are illustrated, except in the case of the cross-table lateral position, which is commonly used for neurological examinations (Fig. 1-1). Unless an expiration film of the lungs is desired, the patient is asked to take a deep breath and hold it for a few seconds. Holding the breath prevents movement of the body and is necessary when taking many types of radiographs of the head, chest, and abdomen to improve the quality of the radiograph.

Posterior. When the term posterior or posterior-anterior (PA) is used, it refers to the x-ray beam penetrating the body from the back (posterior) to the front (anterior). Posterior radiographs are commonly performed in the radiology department. In the case of a chest radiograph, the patient places the anterior side of the chest firmly against a plate or cassette that holds the film. The x-ray machine is positioned 6 feet behind the patient, and the beam penetrates through the patient's back.

Anterior. In some instances, the patient is unable to be transported to the radiology department. In those instances, an anterior-posterior (AP) radiograph may be taken. In the case of a chest radiograph, the patient is usually sitting upright in a bed or lying in a supine position. The x-ray beam is placed approximately 3 feet in front of the patient. The x-ray beam passes through the patient from the anterior to the posterior. Images on an AP chest radiograph are more magnified and less sharp than on a PA film, but the technique has many uses in neuroradiology.

Lateral. A lateral film positions the patient seated or standing, with one side of the body against the x-ray film. For a chest radiograph, the left side of the chest is usually placed next to the x-ray film, and the patient is asked to lock hands behind the back to pull the shoulder blades posteriorly. (Alternately, the patient may reach up and hold a bar or lock arms over the head to move the shoulder blades out of the way.) In this position, the x-ray

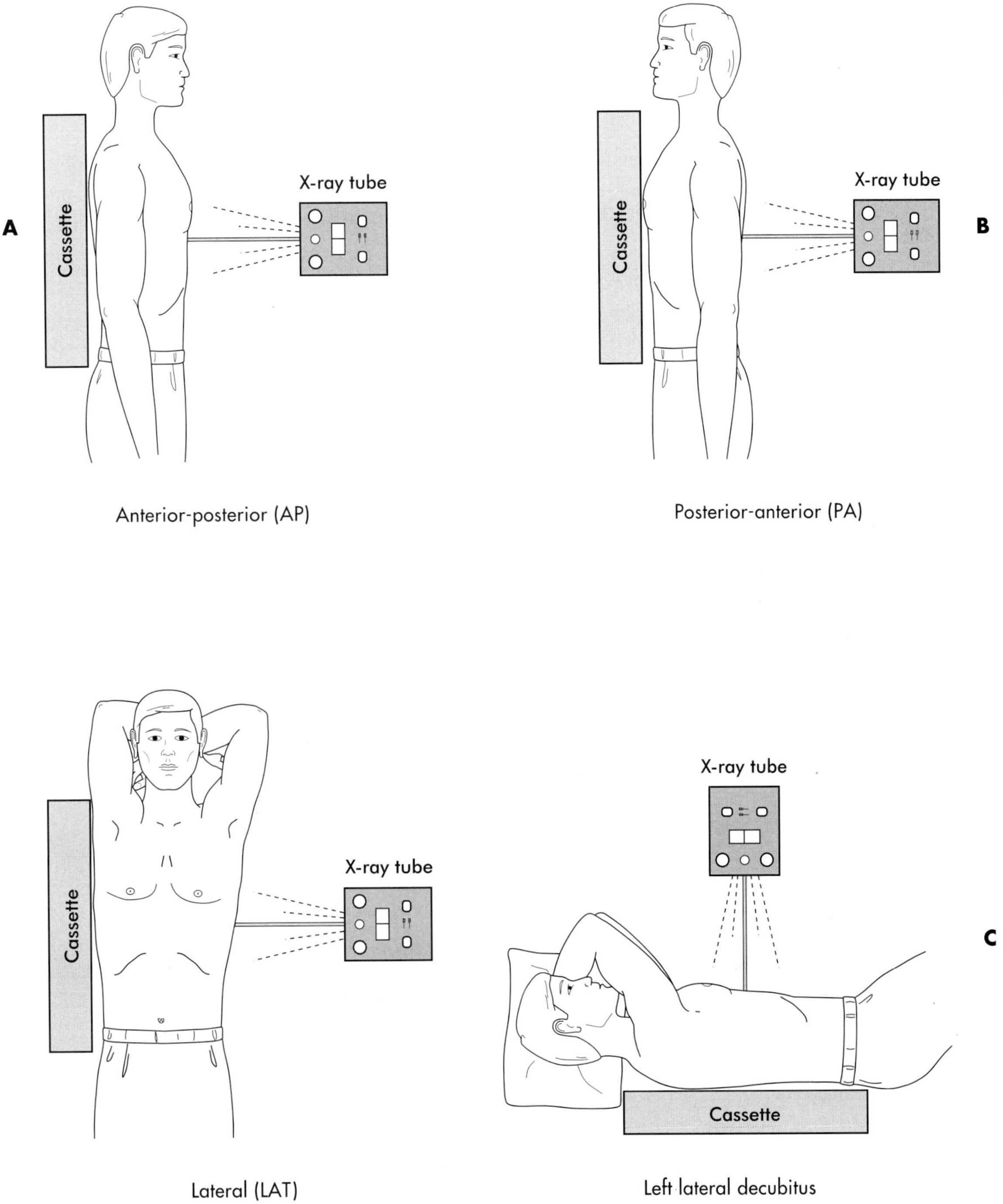

Fig. 1-1 Relative positions of the patient, x-ray cassette, and x-ray beam for **A,** anterior-posterior (AP), **B,** posterior-anterior (PA), and **C,** lateral decubitus positions.

beam passes through the patient from right to left. The physician usually orders a lateral chest radiograph to help identify abnormalities behind the heart, along the spine, or at the base of the lung. A right lateral chest radiograph is ordered when the abnormality, such as a tumor, is in the right lung because images in the right lung are then less magnified and more sharp.

Cross-Table Lateral. In the critical care unit, the skull, spine, or lungs are examined with a radiograph termed *cross-table lateral*. The patient is in a supine position with the head of the bed flat. The patient's shoulders are positioned level with the bed and each other, and the patient's face is directed toward the ceiling. For example, to examine the skull, the film is supported upright next to the patient, above the shoulders and next to the ears, and the x-ray beam is positioned perpendicular to the film.

Lateral Decubitus. For a lateral decubitus radiograph the patient is in a recumbent position, lying on the side. Ideally, the body is not rotated forward or backward. The x-ray film is supported upright next to the patient, and the x-ray beam is directed perpendicular to the film. This technique helps to assess fluid and air levels in the pleural or peritoneal cavities. Fluid flows by way of gravity to the most dependent region and air rises to superior areas.

Oblique. An oblique radiograph allows the body to be seen at an angle. An oblique radiograph of the chest is used to see the trachea or to localize anterior from posterior lesions without interference from bony or overlying structures. A right oblique film places the patient's right anterior side of the chest against the film, and a left oblique film places the left anterior side of the chest against the film.

Lordotic. A lordotic radiograph of the lungs is used to identify apical abnormalities. In a lordotic view, either the patient or the x-ray machine is positioned at a 45-degree angle. This position elevates the clavicle above the apices and also provides a better view of the right and left middle lung fields.

Technique. Specific techniques of penetration and exposure are not covered in this text. Many variables exist that affect the radiograph. These include the type of electrical current available (single or three-phase), the kilowatt rating of the generator and tube, the radiation characteristics (wavelength), the filtration used, the type of film, the type of screens, the grid, and the type of processor and processing solutions. However, it is important for the nurse to understand how differences in exposure affect the radiograph.

Patient Size. Patient size plays a major role in correctly positioning the patient and in choosing appropriate exposure settings. Radiologists classify patients into four body types, beginning with the largest build and progressing to the very slim: hypersthenic, sthenic, hyposthenic, and asthenic. *Hypersthenic* patients are very large and comprise about 5% of the population. The thorax is broad and deep, the diaphragm is high (short lungs), and the abdomen is long. The abdominal organs, especially the stomach, gallbladder, and colon, are usually in a higher position than normal. *Sthenic* patients are a smaller modification of hypersthenic patient and comprise about 50% of the population. The *hyposthenic* patient is more slender than the sthenic, and the *asthenic* patient is of extremely slender build. In the latter the thorax is long, the diaphragm is low, and the abdominal cavity is short (Ballinger, 1991).

Exposure. Ideally, all radiographs of the patient are made in the radiology department with the patient in perfect position and with ideal exposure. In practice, patients may be unable to be transported to the radiology department or they may be less than fully cooperative for positioning. The ability of technologists to accurately predict and accommodate all factors to produce an ideal radiograph is limited. This combination of factors produces films which can hamper assessment.

It is beyond the scope of this text to identify all consequences of incorrect positioning. The nurse must keep in mind that any rotation of the body to the left or right is actually an oblique projection. Assisting the technologist to position the patient and assisting the patient to maintain the appropriate position improves the quality of the radiograph (see Chapter 2).

When a radiograph is overexposed or overpenetrated, structures appear to be darker because too much energy was used to imprint the film. Overexposure occurs more often in patients with an asthenic build. Occasionally overexposure is desirable, but it is often unwanted and makes assessment of films difficult. When comparing structures on an ideal and an overexposed radiograph, fluid-filled structures on the overexposed radiograph may not be apparent. For example, pulmonary edema or infiltrates may not be easily visible.

The opposite of overexposure is underexposure or underpenetration. Underexposure is more common in patients with large muscle or fat masses. With underexposure, insufficient energy is applied to penetrate body tissues.

Compared to an ideal radiograph, black or air-filled areas appear less black and more gray to white and white fluid-filled areas appear even whiter. Even very small fluid-filled vessels are visible. It is easy to overassess fluid overload states and infiltrates in an underpenetrated film.

If the nurse must compare an overpenetrated radiograph with an underpenetrated radiograph, it is important to compare the intensity of the change on one radiograph to the intensity of the change on the second radiograph. The nurse should measure the size of the affected area on both films to determine if the involved area has increased, decreased, or stayed the same size. The nurse may also compare the relative whiteness or blackness of the area to surrounding structures on the film. A physician or technologist can help the nurse to appreciate differences in penetration/exposure technique.

Densities. There are four primary densities found on a radiograph: metal, fluid/water, fat, and air (Fig. 1-2). Denser tissues absorb more of the x-ray beam than less dense tissues. When a tissue absorbs more radiation, it appears more opaque or white on the radiograph. Conversely, less dense tissues absorb less radiation; they are more radiolucent and appear blacker on a radiograph.

Metals, such as necklaces, electrocardiogram electrodes, fillings in the teeth, coins, bullet fragments or shotgun pellets, appear bright white on a radiograph. Bones, which are rich in calcium, appear slightly less white than dense metals. Fluid/water density is also white on a radiograph, but it is less white than bone or metal. Blood vessels and blood-filled organs like the heart and liver demonstrate fluid/water density on a radiograph. In fluid overload states, more fluid-filled vessels are observed on the radiograph. Fat is less dense, and thus is less white than metals or water. Fat is readily apparent on chest and abdominal films, but rarely seen on skull radiographs. The most common fatty areas seen on a chest radiograph are breast tissue and fat surrounding the rib cage. Abdominal fat is readily visible on the outer borders of abdominal films. Lung tissue is filled with air in the normal lung; it is radiolucent and should appear black on a normal chest x-ray film. Increased radiolucency is a sign of air trapping, as seen in emphysema and asthma. Increased radiopacity or "white-out" of lung fields suggests fluid (e.g., pneumonia or pulmonary edema) or tumor.

Film Labeling

Various labels are applied to the radiograph by the technologist. The purpose of the labels is to permanently identify the radiograph for future review and

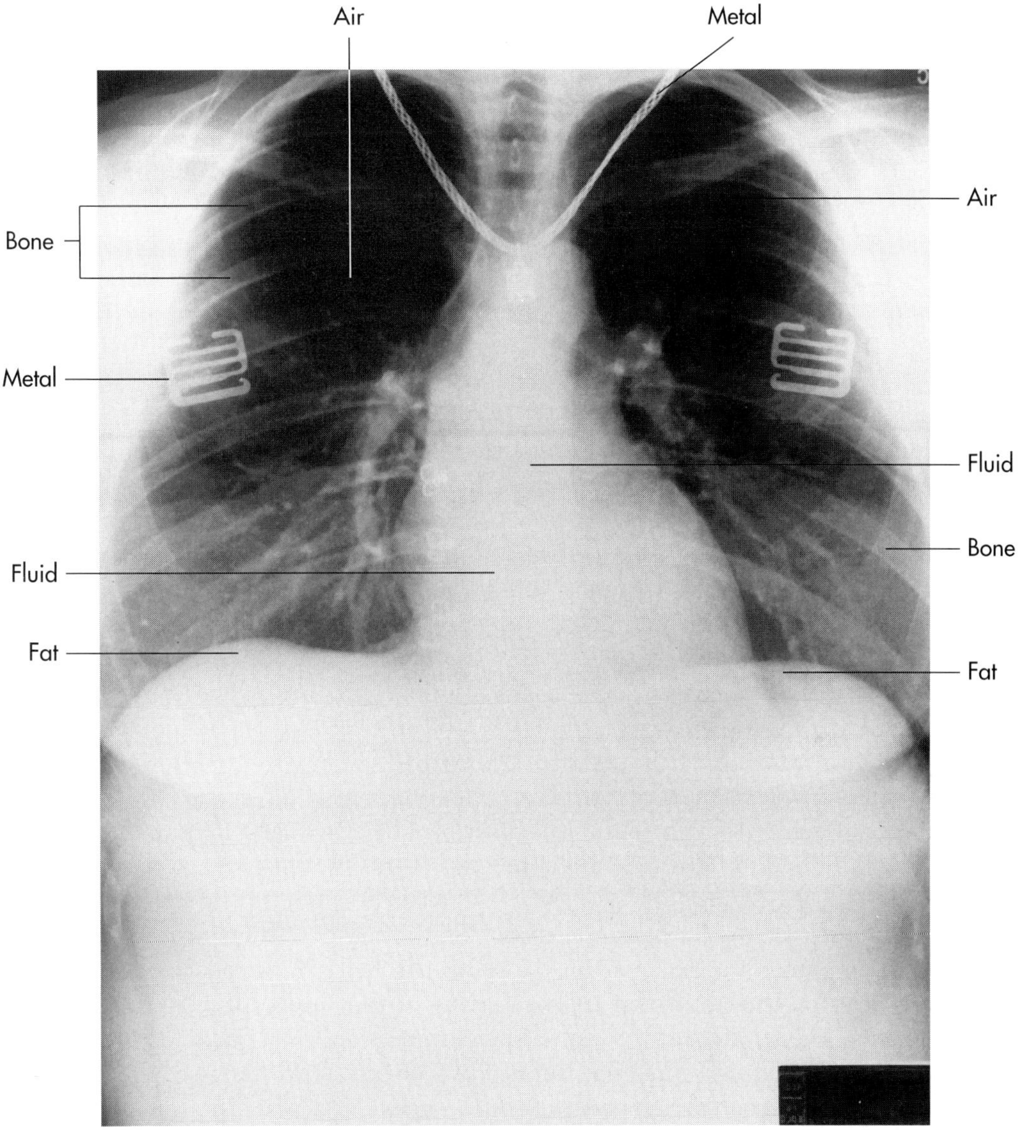

Fig. 1-2 Densities on a radiograph include metal (the brightest white or radiopaque), bone, which contains calcium (slightly less white or radiopaque than metal), blood vessels like the heart, which is fluid or water density (less radiopaque than metal), fat (even less radiopaque than metal or fluid), and air (radiolucent or black).

comparison. A corner of the radiograph contains information pertinent to patient identification such as name, age or date of birth, medical record or case number, or attending physician. This information is necessary because there may be multiple John Smiths having radiographs taken at the same institution; the patient's birth date, age, or medical record number helps identify the correct patient. The radiograph also contains the date (and possibly the time) the test was performed and the name of the institution.

Markers are generally applied to the radiograph by the technologist that indicate right, left, up, down, or patient position (e.g., decubitus, upright, or supine). There are time markers in studies involving injection of contrast or depth markers for special examinations, such as the CT scan. The labels are often metallic and may be applied in the darkroom or secured to the outside of the x-ray cassette just before exposure. When metallic imprint markers are not used, pertinent information is written directly on the film after processing or a sticker containing the information is secured to the film. Occasionally the marker, such as an arrow or a dot, is applied to the patient's skin and radiographs are exposed using different techniques or patient positions. The marker is used as a reference point when the radiologist interprets the film; this technique is useful in identifying position of tumors or foreign bodies.

Types of X-rays. Conventional radiographs are primarily discussed in this text, with few exceptions. There are other imaging techniques available that are intermittently used in the critical care patient. These techniques include ventilation-perfusion scans, angiography, CT scans, MRI and PET scans. Each type of radiograph is discussed briefly to provide the nurse with a foundation for differences in technology.

Ventilation-Perfusion Scans. Ventilation-perfusion scan is one type of nuclear medicine method for imaging the body. The most common scans ordered by the physician include scans of the brain, lungs, thyroid, liver, spleen, kidney, heart, and bone. Each organ requires a particular radioactive isotope for optimal imaging. Radioactive particles are inhaled into the lungs or administered intravenously, and a specialized machine (gas detector or scintillator) counts the decay of the radioactive particles. For instance, a radioactive xenon or technetium compound is used to examine the exchange of oxygen and carbon dioxide in the lungs, and an iodine compound is used for the liver. In the case of the lungs, either a ventilation scan, a perfusion scan, or both can be performed at one time. Ventilation scans are difficult to perform in patients who are receiving continuous mechanical ventilation.

Angiography. Angiograms record the progressive flow of a contrast material through a blood vessel in a series of radiographs that are exposed from fractions of a second to seconds apart. In the critically ill patient, angiograms are commonly performed to identify carotid, vertebral, thoracic or abdominal aortic aneurysm, or pulmonary embolism. Where appropriate, angiograms are shown in the text.

Computed Tomography. Computed tomography (CT) is a term used to describe a technique commercially developed in the late 1960s that produces a cross-sectional image or "slice" of a section of the body. The image is reconstructed by a computer using x-ray absorption measurements around the scanned area. Body parts are not overlapping as in standard radiographic projections; body parts above and below the cut section are eliminated from the picture. Sequential cuts at predetermined distances essentially build a three-dimensional image of the patient on a two-dimensional film.

Magnetic Resonance Imaging. Like CT scanning, MRI is a computer-based cross-sectional imaging technique, but it does not use any ionizing radiation. Instead, MRI uses the interactions of electromagnetic forces and body tissues to produce images. MRI is not portable and has limited use in the critical care patient. It is beyond the scope of this text to discuss assessment of MRI films.

Positron Emission Tomography. PET scanning is a noninvasive imaging technique that is predominantly used to measure cellular, organ, or systemic function, including blood flow and metabolism. It requires administration of a radiopharmaceutical and produces a functional image of the body part being examined through positron-electron annihilation. Since PET is still in the research phase and is rarely used in the critical care setting, it will not be covered further in this text.

REFERENCE

Ballinger PW: *Merrill's Atlas of radiographic positions and radiologic procedures,* ed 7, St Louis, 1991, Mosby.

2 Nursing Responsibilities

OBTAINING A QUALITY FILM

The nurse is responsible for many of the components involved in obtaining a radiograph. The nurse may be involved in scheduling the test by telephone or computer. In order to not delay testing and obtain the best quality film, the nurse should ask about special test requirements when scheduling the test or consult the radiographic procedure manual. The nurse should also inform the radiology department about special patient needs, such as oxygen, mechanical ventilation, gastric tubes, or invasive catheters.

Often it is the bedside nurse who educates the patient about the test to be performed. Some institutions have a nurse who specializes in radiographic procedures and is active in patient education. Most radiographic examinations require some kind of preparation, even in the intensive care unit. At a minimum, the x-ray cassette is positioned behind the body part to be radiographed. The technologist or the nurse should explain to the patients the position they will need to assume and maintain. In many instances the position is uncomfortable; patients may complain of pain from surgical or traumatic wounds when they are moved to position the x-ray cassette. Some patients will require administration of analgesics or sedatives before lengthy or painful radiographic procedures. For all radiographs, the patient must remain motionless during the time the film is being exposed to the x-ray beam. Motion produces distortion and can make the radiograph impossible to interpret.

There are several simple actions that improve the quality of an x-ray film (see the box on p. 14). In a critical situation it is easy to overlook some of them, especially repositioning lines and patient privacy. The lines can obscure important structures such as lung infiltrates, and a patient worried about exposure of private body parts may be tense and difficult to position.

TIPS TO IMPROVE X-RAY FILM QUALITY

- Remove ornaments or prostheses (necklaces, earrings, hair pins, and removable dental work)
- Secure the patient's removable valuables with tape
- Move the external portions of intravenous, intraarterial, or nasogastric invasive lines, electrocardiograph monitor wires, and oxygen or mechanical ventilator tubings away from the body parts to be radiographed
- Cover the patient's exposed breasts, buttocks, and genitalia; pull the drapes, close the door, or restrict visitors to the unit

The technologist, usually with the nurse's assistance, will position and support the patient with pillows or immobilization devices to prevent muscle strain, keeping in mind what structures need to be viewed. The nurse should follow the directions of the technologist to help position the patient and x-ray cassette. To protect the patient and health care providers, an immobile patient should never be lifted or rolled without assistance and good body mechanics.

The nurse may be required to administer intravenous, nasogastric, or urinary dye contrast material to permit a view of vascular or other structures. A patent intravenous catheter and an ample supply of fluids prevents unnecessary discomfort in the patient. The nurse should make sure the catheter is secured with tape and/or a dressing before positioning the patient for the radiograph. Gastric or duodenal tube feedings may need to be stopped well in advance of some abdominal radiographs.

Many chest radiographs require that the patient either inhale or exhale maximally and hold the breath; others require even, slow breathing. In the case of a patient receiving mechanical ventilation, the exposure of the radiograph must often coincide with the cycling of the ventilator or the nurse must manually inflate the lungs with an AMBU-bag or manual resuscitator to obtain the correct lung inflation. Less often the radiograph is exposed during full exhalation.

A radiation technologist, alone or with a radiologist, takes the radiograph. To obtain a quality test with minimal risk to the patient, the nurse should inform the technologist of pertinent historical and physical examination findings. For instance, if a patient with a cervical spine fracture (or a patient in whom spinal injury has not been ruled out) needs a chest radiograph, the technologist must be told that the patient has a possible neck fracture and must be logrolled to position the x-ray cassette. Other patients may not be able to have the head position altered or to roll in a particular direction. The technologist must be made aware of patients with communicable diseases, secretions, or drainage. In some instances the x-ray cassette may need to be placed in a bag to prevent contamination.

Safety Issues

Some nurses are anxious about radiation exposure. Excessive radiation from any source can cause injury, but there are many techniques nurses can use to promote their own and the patient's safety.

The three main factors that determine radiation exposure are time, distance, and shielding (Ballinger, 1991). Different types of radiographs require different exposure times. The usual plain radiograph taken in the patient's room needs an exposure of approximately 1 second; fluoroscopy for placing invasive catheters usually requires up to 60 seconds of exposure at one time. More radiation exposure is possible with longer exposure times.

Distance, the second factor, is critical in determining radiation exposure. The closer the nurse is to the beam or the field of penetration, the greater the radiation exposure risk becomes. Larger fields of radiation produce wider scattering of ionizing radiation, potentially placing the nurse at greater risk. If the radiation exposure is 100% at a distance of 1 foot from the beam and if it can be halved by moving each additional foot away from the beam, then the nurse can control the level of potential radiation exposure by increasing the distance from the patient. At a distance of 3 to 4 feet, or roughly arm's length from the patient, the potential for radiation exposure is approximately 25% or less of the total patient exposure dose. Increasing the distance from the beam to 6 feet virtually eliminates substantial radiation exposure. In addition, since the nurse is not directly in front of the beam, as is the patient, most of the radiation exposure is from scatter.

Shielding is the third component that determines radiation exposure. Wearing a lead-lined rubber or vinyl apron reduces the risk of radiation exposure to susceptible organs. Most aprons contain 0.5 mm of lead lining in the front of the apron and 0.3 mm in the back. This affords low-to-moderate protection from radiation. Some aprons completely cover the chest, sides, and back of the nurse or contain a thyroid shield; these aprons should be used by nurses who are involved with fluoroscopy or other procedures with sustained risk of radiation exposure. Since cracks in the lead reduce the amount of protection from radiation exposure, care should be taken to maintain the integrity of the lead lining. The lead apron should be hung over a wide bar or on a specially-designed hanger after use; it should never be folded or dropped onto the floor. With care, a lead apron should protect the nurse against radiation for approximately 10 years.

It is important to know how much radiation exposure critical care nurses encounter while performing their duties. Many institutions require nurses to wear radiation exposure badges to determine the level of radiation exposure. The badge should be worn outside the lead apron in a conspicuous area, usually by the collar to determine the amount of radiation to the thyroid or on the belt to determine gonadal radiation. The badge should be applied at the start of the nursing shift and removed at the end of the shift. Badges are replaced monthly and sent for a reading of radiation exposure levels. Nurses who exceed safe levels of radiation exposure should either review safety protection measures or have their assignment changed.

Assessing the Radiograph

Depending on the type of critical care unit nurses work in their duties do not end with taking the radiograph. In some institutions the nurse provides the initial assessment of the x-ray film, and in others the x-ray film is delivered to the critical care unit or the patient's room. Just as the nurse is not a cardiologist interpreting electrocardiograms, the nurse is not a radiologist and is not expected to interpret the radiograph. The nurse should use the radiograph as another assessment parameter like the electrocardiogram, which is used to validate clinical assessment parameters or suspected pathology. As shown in the following few examples, the nurse should always tie anatomical findings on the radiograph to clinical findings. It is imperative that the nurse be familiar with normal anatomy.

Perhaps the nurse assesses crackles in a particular lung field; the chest radiograph is assessed for atelectasis or infiltrates in that area. Similarly, dullness to percussion should be correlated with pleural effusion or lung collapse. An enlarging abdomen should be correlated to bowel gas, excessive stool, fluid layering from bleeding, or other possibilities. If a nurse assesses loss of motor function in the lower or upper extremities, the cervical or thoracic spine films or computerized tomography (CT) scan of the head should be assessed for abnormalities or worsening of the existing problem.

When assessing the radiograph, the nurse needs to use a consistent process for analysis. An individual's technique may vary, but each nurse should develop a systematic approach that is used every time a radiograph is assessed. The nurse first analyzes the quality of the film and then assesses anatomical structures. Whenever possible, the nurse should compare the current film to a previous one. Sometimes differences in penetration or positioning make comparison difficult; this is especially true in anterior-posterior (AP) films of the chest or abdomen that are taken in the critical care unit.

A good method of routinely and completely scrutinizing the radiograph is to assess it as you would the patient's body: always moving from external to internal, side to side, and top to bottom. For example, when examining a radiograph, the nurse should first scrutinize the soft tissue area, the bony structures, inner layers just under the bones, and finally the internal structures like the cerebral hemispheres, lungs, heart, or abdominal viscera. If this pattern is followed consistently, it will be difficult to miss obvious or even obscure abnormalities.

What should the nurse do if possible abnormality is identified? The nurse should always confirm the finding with a qualified physician. In teaching institutions, the resident may be contacted for preliminary interpretation. While awaiting final confirmation, the nurse should prepare for anticipated orders such as chest tube, intracranial catheter, or tong insertion.

In some instances, locating the position of an abnormality may directly impact nursing care. For example, if the nurse assesses an infiltrate in the left lower lung field, postural drainage including chest percussion would be more effectively directed to the affected area. Positioning may also be used to drain pleural effusions or pneumothoraces, or to enhance feeding tube migration.

In summary, taking a radiography is a common occurrence in an intensive care unit. With proper patient preparation by the nurse and radiation technologist team, a quality radiograph can be produced. Even in the most critical situations, nurses should remember to protect themselves and the patient from excessive radiation and to consult the physician for accurate interpretation of the radiograph.

REFERENCE

Ballinger PW: *Merrill's Atlas of radiographic positions and radiologic procedures,* ed 7, St Louis, 1991, Mosby.

3 Assessment of the Patient
Chest Radiography

The standard radiograph of the chest is a posterior-anterior (PA) projection, usually accompanied by a lateral projection. In the intensive care unit the conventional radiograph is an anterior-posterior (AP) portable chest film. Lateral decubitus radiographs are frequently ordered to identify presence, loculation, and magnitude of pleural effusions. The physician will occasionally order a lordotic radiograph to examine the apices; more commonly, however, the physician receives a lordotic radiograph without request because of inadequate positioning of the patient and x-ray beam. Oblique radiographs are rarely ordered unless the trachea must be viewed. An oblique radiograph is also useful in differentiating anterior from posterior lesions in the presence of bilateral lung disease.

NORMAL STRUCTURES

Knowledge of the normal anatomy of the lung is essential in order to properly assess a chest radiograph. The nurse must know the position of the ribs and clavicle, the location of the pleura, and the structures of the lung, airways, and heart. Each of these areas is briefly reviewed in the order in which they should be assessed on the chest radiograph (Fig. 3-1).

Soft Tissue

The lungs are completely encased in the bony thorax, which is covered with skin and soft tissues. When examining the skin and soft tissues, the nurse should assess for depth and homogeneity of soft tissue, beginning with lateral areas and moving medially. Lack of homogeneity is usually abnormal. Air

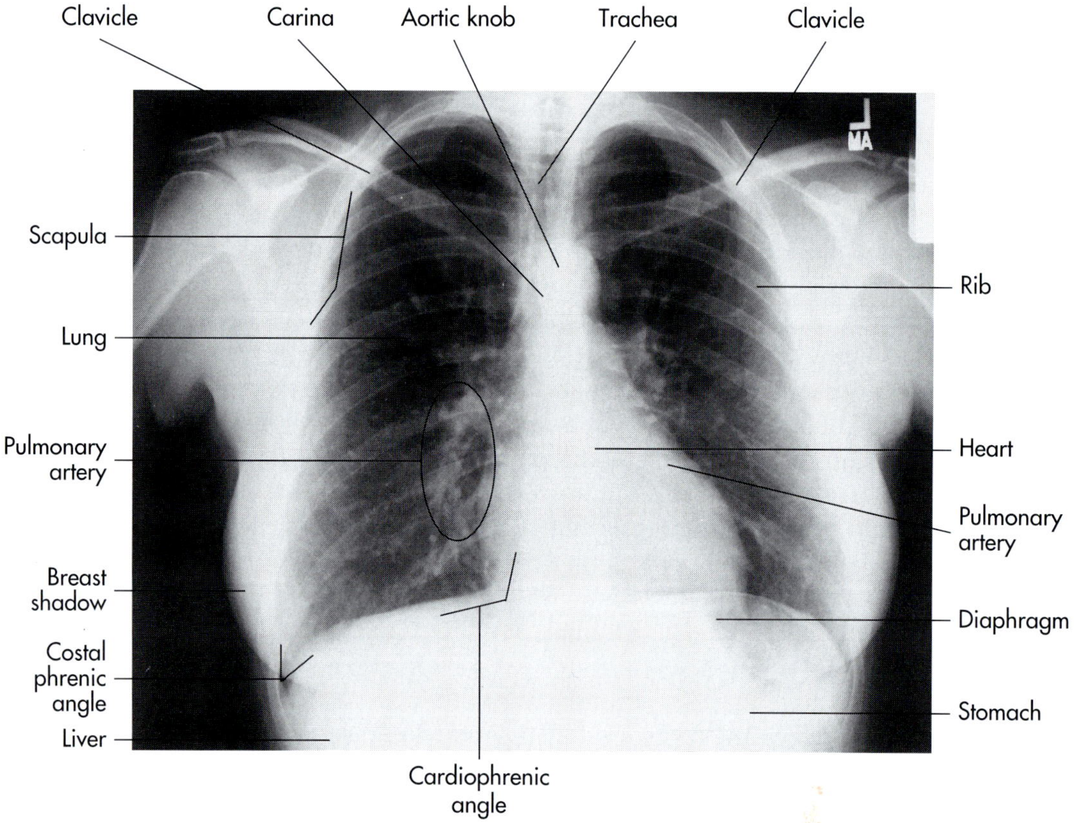

Fig. 3-1 Normal position of anatomical structures on a posterior or anterior chest radiograph.

(subcutaneous emphysema) seen in the lateral soft tissues suggests the presence of a pneumothorax. Overlapping densities suggest fluid accumulation, skin folds, or possibly postoperative changes. Breast shadows and rarely the nipple area are evident on a chest film. Unilateral absence of breast tissue, such as that seen with a full or partial mastectomy patient can make one lung appear more radiolucent and one lung more radiopaque.

Bony Structures

The bony structures in the chest include the ribs, clavicles, sternum, manubrium, spine, and vertebrae. The nurse counts the ribs, starting at the top and working down. Approximately 8 to 9 ribs should overlie lung tissue on an inspiratory chest film. If fewer than 8 ribs overlie lung tissue, a poor inspiration or small lung volumes are suggested. While counting the ribs the nurse should follow the curve of each rib from the anterior around posteriorly to the spine. In a well-penetrated chest radiograph, the viewer can count the thoracic vertebrae as well as the ribs, allowing identification of obvious fractures or the absence of rib segments or a complete rib. A rib may be partially removed during surgical procedures, or cancers may obliterate rib segments.

The nurse examines the chest film for position and to check that the clavicles, which are usually located at the second or third intercostal space, are intact. The heads (medial portions) of the clavicles should be centered exactly over the posterior vertebral column (spine). If the clavicular heads are not in this position, the patient and the beam were not correctly aligned and the film is said to be rotated, making the film slightly oblique. Rotation of the patient can dramatically alter assessment of fluid status and infiltrates.

The scapulae, like the ribs and clavicles, are assessed for correct position and intactness. Often the posterior scapulae are mistaken for a pneumothorax, especially on an AP film. This is one reason the PA chest radiograph is more desirable—the shoulders are rotated forward, pulling the scapulae apart. This error can be avoided by looking for lung markings past the scapular line.

Pleura and Diaphragm

There are two pleurae in the chest: the visceral pleura, covering each lobe of the lung, and the parietal pleura, near the rib side. The parietal and visceral pleurae are separated by a potential space containing about 25 ml of fluid to prevent friction as the lungs expand and contract. Each lobe of the lung is separated by an interlobar fissure, which can be seen on a quality chest radiograph. The major fissure separates the upper and lower lobes and runs obliquely from posterior to anterior, beginning approximately at the level of the fifth thoracic vertebra and extending down to the diaphragm. The major fissure is usually not visible on a PA projection because it is not parallel to the x-ray beam; it is best seen on a lateral chest radiograph.

The right upper and middle lobes are separated by the minor fissure. When visible the minor fissure is seen in both PA and lateral x-ray films, but it is not apparent on the chest films of 44% of all adult patients (Felson, 1965, 1973). The minor fissure extends from the anterior chest wall and intersects the major fissure on a lateral chest radiograph. Usually seen at approximately the level of the fourth rib, the minor fissure may appear as high as the second or as low as the sixth rib. The lower the minor fissure, the smaller the right middle lobe. The nurse should learn the correct positions of the fissures on a chest radiograph. Displacement of the fissure from normal position on a chest x-ray film often indicates the presence of lobar collapse. Atelectasis, or collapse of a segment or lobe, pulls the fissure toward the collapsed area.

The nurse assesses the contour of the diaphragm. A normally-shaped diaphragm is rounded, with sharp, pointed costophrenic angles. The cardiophrenic (medial) angle is slightly less sharp than the costophrenic angle. The right diaphragm is usually 1 to 2 cm higher than the left. The dome of the diaphragm is frequently identified at the level of the sixth rib. Blunting of the costophrenic or cardiophrenic angle suggests pleural effusion. A lower or flatter diaphragm suggests hyperinflation, which occurs in emphysema.

Lungs

The lung parenchyma, next to the pleura, is assessed next. The nurse compares the right and left sides from top to bottom, as in chest assessment. The lungs contain air and should be radiolucent or appear black or dark compared to the fluid-filled heart and the bones. The trachea, generally seen in the midline over the thoracic vertebrae, also contains air and is radiolucent. The nurse should suspect an abnormality if there are diffuse or localized areas of increased radiopacity (whiteness) or increased translucency (blackness).

If diffuse increased radiopacity is identified by the nurse, it may be classified as an alveolar pattern, an interstitial pattern, or a vascular pattern; each of which is associated with different pathology. Fluffy, soft, poorly demarcated opacifications that are usually less than 1 cm in diameter define an alveolar pattern. As the alveoli fill with water density material, the normal vascular pattern is clouded. The nurse may observe air bronchograms with an alveolar pattern. Normally, airways other than the trachea are not visible on a chest radiograph. If the airway is surrounded by fluid, the outline of the bronchus appears on the chest radiograph. This phenomenon is termed *air bronchogram* and implies consolidation of fluid around the airway. The most common cause of an alveolar pattern on chest x-ray film is cardiogenic or non-cardiogenic pulmonary edema, although it is also associated with other causes such as viral pneumonia, pneumocystis, and alveolar cell carcinoma.

Consolidation of interstitial tissue (including alveolar walls, intralobular vessels, interlobar septa, and connective tissue) surrounding the pulmonary vessels and bronchial tree causes an interstitial pattern. A branching line with multiple thin strands that radiate toward the periphery of the lung characterizes an interstitial pattern. These lines may intersect to form a network and are often referred to as *Kerley lines*. The most common causes of an interstitial pattern on a chest radiograph are pulmonary fibrosis and interstitial pneumonitis. Physicians recognize interstitial lung diseases by the appearance of honeycombs (multiple, round translucent areas surrounded by dense interstitial consolidations) that range in size up to 1 cm.

Vascular patterns are the third type of lung marking and are useful for identifying left ventricular failure, pulmonary hypertension, and emphysema. Vascular patterns are derived from the pulmonary arteries and their vast capillary network.

The nurse assesses the hilar area for position and size. The right hilum is usually no more than 2 cm lower than the left hilum, which is just below the aortic knob. An enlarged left or right hilum is not uncommon in lung cancer with lymph node involvement. The nurse traces the pulmonary vessels from the hila out to the periphery. The pulmonary arteries typically decrease in size from their trunk in the hilum to the periphery. An increase in the size of the pulmonary arteries in the hilum as they extend out into the lung is associated with pulmonary hypertension. An isolated decrease in the size, truncation, or obliteration of a pulmonary artery is associated with a large pulmonary embolus. In the periphery of the lung, blood vessels appear as tiny lines, almost imperceptible even up close and under normal conditions. Enlarged pulmonary vessels near the periphery are associated with left ventricular failure and fluid overload. Cephalization, an increase in the prominence of the apical vessels, is usually observed in congestive heart failure. Lack of vascular marking in the periphery suggests the presence of a pneumothorax. Pulmonary stenosis and emphysema are associated with a general decrease in vascular markings in the lung.

Cardiac Structures

The nurse also assesses the appearance of the mediastinum, which sits in the midline of the body between the lungs. The heart, shaped somewhat like a cone, is about 12 cm long, 9 cm wide, and 6 cm deep. It sits obliquely toward the left in the middle mediastinum. The apex of the heart, which sits on the diaphragm and against the anterior wall of the chest, is directed anteriorly, inferiorly, to the left; the base of the heart extends posteriorly, superiorly, and to the right. When the heart extends more into the left side of the chest, ventricular enlargement or cardiomegaly is present. With cardiomegaly the heart may also extend into the right side of the chest. To determine whether enlargement of the heart is present, the nurse compares its width to that of a hemithorax using a ruler or finger span. The heart is said to be enlarged when it occupies space equivalent to more than one third of a hemithorax in a PA film or one half of an AP film.

The nurse also inspects the chest radiograph for abnormalities in position or size of the large vessels, for mediastinal widening, especially at the level of the aortic knob, and for the presence of air or calcium in the mediastinum. Listed below are common findings on the chest radiograph of an ICU patient.

ATELECTASIS

Definition

Atelectasis is the collapse of the alveoli from obstruction, compression, or contraction. The obstruction may be central, such as from aspiration of foreign body or from tumor, or peripheral, such as from postoperative atelectasis or from mucus related to pneumonia. Compression atelectasis develops from external pressure or squeezing on the alveoli, often the result of a pneumothorax or pleural effusion. Contraction atelectasis results from scarring that causes a decrease in lung volume, which can occur with tuberculosis, silicosis, or pulmonary fibrosis.

Clinical Findings

Although many patients are asymptomatic, some may have fever and chest tightness. Patients may complain of chest pain, especially with large areas of collapse. On inspection the nurse may observe dyspnea, tachypnea, tracheal deviation, or cyanosis. Palpation is often not revealing, but there may be tactile fremitus. With large areas of collapse, dullness to percussion is observed. The nurse may find crackles, wheezes, or decreased breath sounds with auscultation.

Radiologic Appearance

Areas of atelectasis appear more dense or radiopaque on the x-ray film (Fig. 3-2). The term *plate-like atelectasis* is used to describe saucer-shaped areas of atelectasis. To identify atelectasis, the nurse must first identify proper placement of the fissures, hilum (including the trachea), and mediastinum, because displacement is often related to collapse. Lobar or multisegmental collapse causes these structures to be pulled *toward* the area of atelectasis. Unilateral atelectasis sometimes elevates the diaphragm on the side of collapse; however, the right diaphragm is usually slightly higher. In some cases the distance between the ribs narrows and an air bronchogram may be present. An air bronchogram is air that shows through a greater density such as water or mucus. Bronchi are not usually seen on the x-ray film because they are thin-walled, contain air, and are surrounded by alveolar air. When multiple air bronchograms are crowded together, there is usually segmental or lobar collapse. An air bronchogram is present only when the airway contains air and the surrounding tissue does not. Bronchi that are filled with secretions do not appear as an air bronchogram but as an infiltrate. Also, air bronchograms only occur when airways are involved; they do not occur when there is an extrapulmonary abnormality such as pleural, mediastinal, or chest wall disease because these structures do not contain air-filled bronchi. (See also the discussion on infiltrates for information on locating areas of involvement.)

Nursing Implications

When atelectasis is diagnosed, it is important to encourage the patient to breathe deeply to reexpand the alveoli and expel the mucus or foreign body. Chest physical therapy or internal percussion may be needed. If a tumor is the cause of atelectasis, the patient may undergo chemotherapy, radiation, or surgery to relieve the obstruction. If mucus is retained, an infection may develop (bronchitis or pneumonia) and the patient may require antibiotics. Judicious pain control (controlling pain without depressing respirations) for deep breathing and coughing is necessary in the postoperative patient.

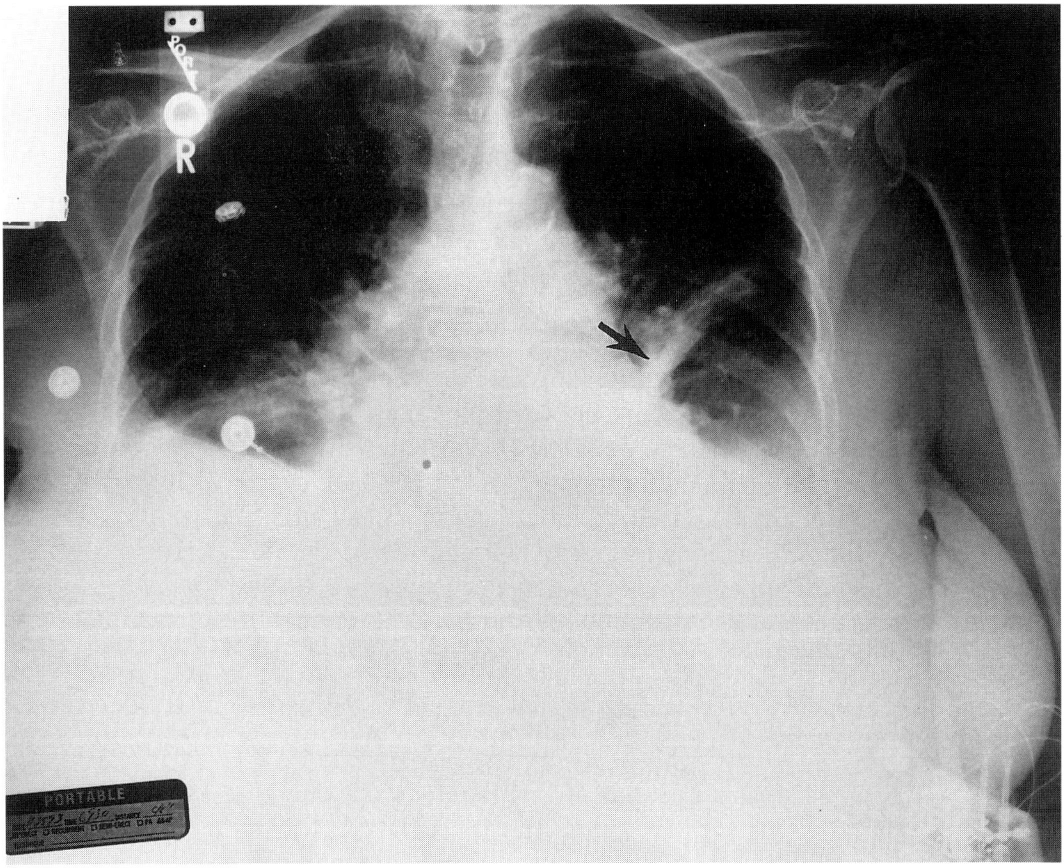

Fig. 3-2 Notice the increased density of atelectasis in the left middle lung field.

AUTOMATIC IMPLANTABLE CARDIAC DEFIBRILLATOR

Definition

An automatic implantable cardiac defibrillator (AICD) is inserted in the patient with recurrent, lethal, ventricular dysrhythmias that are unresponsive to medication. When the device senses ventricular tachycardia or ventricular fibrillation, it delivers a preset amount of electrical pulse directly to the heart muscle. In many instances the ventricular dysrhythmia reverts to a sinus or other preexisting rhythm.

Clinical Findings

The patient who requires an AICD has usually undergone electrophysiology stimulation testing and has been found to have refractory ventricular dysrhythmias, which greatly increases the risk of sudden death. During periods of normal rhythms the patient is totally functional. The patient may be awake or unconscious when ventricular dysrhythmias occur.

Radiologic Appearance

An AICD has one or two flyswatter-like metal patches that are applied over the myocardium, and one to two sensing leads that are placed on the left atrium, right ventricle, or left ventricle. The chest radiograph has the appearance of metallic spaghetti, but the nurse can usually identify one or two semi-rectangular shapes in the mediastinum near the diaphragm. The rectangles are not true in shape because the patches must conform to the myocardium. The sensing leads look like pacing wires. All of the metal wires descend through the diaphragm to the AICD box (Fig. 3-3).

Nursing Implications

Nursing implications are similar to those for patients with pacemakers (see page 57). In addition, if one of the wires becomes displaced, the nurse may observe an enlarging pericardium and tamponade physiology.

A

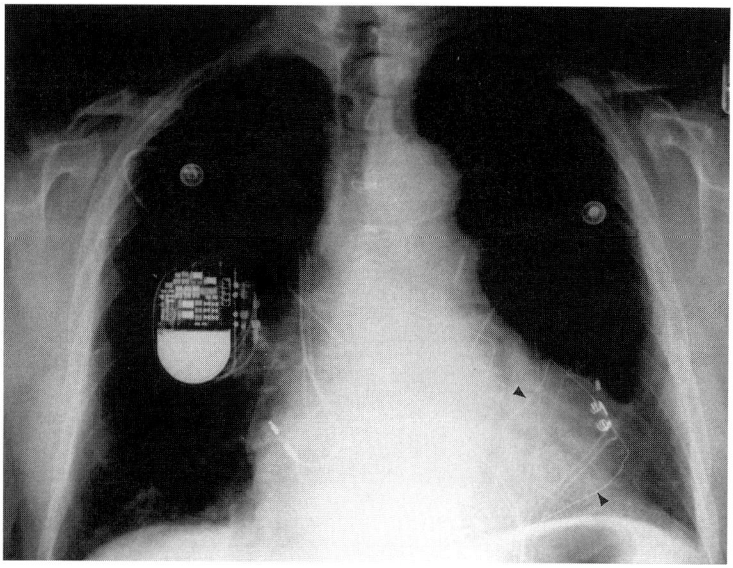

B

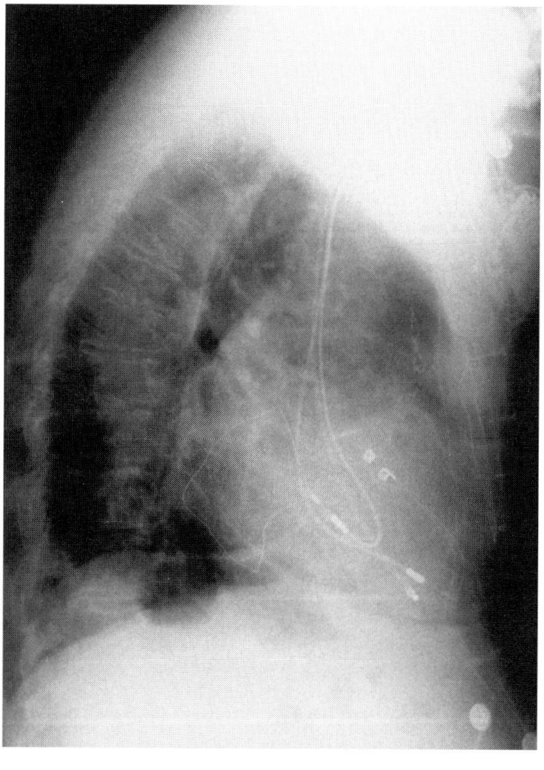

Fig. 3-3 Note the position of the flyswatter patches of an AICD on the **A,** anterior and **B,** lateral radiographs. This patient also has a pacemaker in place.

CENTRAL VEIN CATHETERS

Definition

Invasive central vein catheters are frequently required in the critically or chronically ill patient for administration of fluids, nutrition, medications, and blood products. Central vein catheters are most often inserted through the subclavian or jugular vein, but the femoral vein may provide emergency access at times. Most central vein catheters are approximately 8 inches in length and are inserted percutaneously. Some permanent catheters, such as Porta-cath or Infusa-port, are inserted surgically and have no external infusion ports; others, like the Hickman, have an external and an internal catheter component that can be seen on the chest radiograph. The positioning for temporary and permanent catheters is the same.

Clinical Findings

Temporary catheters have an external component; permanent catheters may not have a visible port. Permanent catheters without a visible port can be palpated just under the skin in the clavicular area. Unless infection is present, the area should be free of redness, swelling, and exudative drainage.

Radiologic Appearance

The nurse can identify the origin and position of a central venous catheter on a chest radiograph. When the central venous catheter is inserted through the internal jugular vein, the nurse observes a thin radiopaque line extending from near the jaw into the superior vena cava. If the central venous catheter originates in the subclavian vein, a thin line that lies under the clavicle and extends into the superior vena cava may be observed. In some very rare cases, the nurse may observe the tip of the catheter extending upward toward the head; in this instance the nurse should alert the physician for prompt removal and reinsertion. If the catheter has been inserted through the femoral vein, the nurse should identify the tip of the catheter in the inferior vena cava; it will appear as if the catheter is coming through the diaphragm. The tip of any central venous catheter should not extend into the right atrium. Since there is always a risk for pneumothorax with insertion of a central venous catheter, particularly with the subclavian vein approach, the nurse should always look for a pneumothorax. When a Hickman catheter is inserted, the nurse observes a thick line extending into the superior vena cava from a subclavian vein. Because the catheter tunnels subcutaneously to the lower rib cage or upper abdomen, the nurse can see the catheter on the chest radiograph; it is usually a vertical line extending down the hemithorax from the subclavian insertion point (Figs. 3-4, 3-5, and 3-6).

Nursing Implications

In the critically ill patient, the nurse is concerned with the proper placement of invasive lines. Although the physician always determines proper placement of invasive lines and tubings, the nurse should be familiar with proper placement to alert the physician and prevent serious complications. Fluids, medications, and blood products should generally not be infused until placement is verified.

CHEST TUBES

Definition

A chest tube is a small- or large-bore flexible plastic catheter or tube that is inserted in the pleural space or mediastinum to remove air (pneumothorax), to facilitate drainage of fluids (pleural effusion, hemothorax, empyema, chylothorax), and to prevent air or fluid from reentering the chest. The chest tube may be angled or straight and made of vinyl, silastic, or latex nonthrombogenic material. The length of the chest tube varies with its size; some physicians may further shorten the tube during insertion to meet patient needs. After insertion, the chest tube is connected to a drainage system or duck-bill valve device that allows aseptic accumulation of fluids and evacuation of air.

Clinical Findings

Patients who require chest tubes may have a variety of clinical findings, including asymmetry of movement (pneumothorax or effusion), dullness to percussion (effusion), crackles just above an effusion, decreased breath sounds (effusion or pneumothorax), or hyperresonance (pneumothorax). After the chest tube is inserted, the nurse may hear a pleural friction rub over the chest tube. The nurse may also palpate crepitus in the skin near the chest tube.

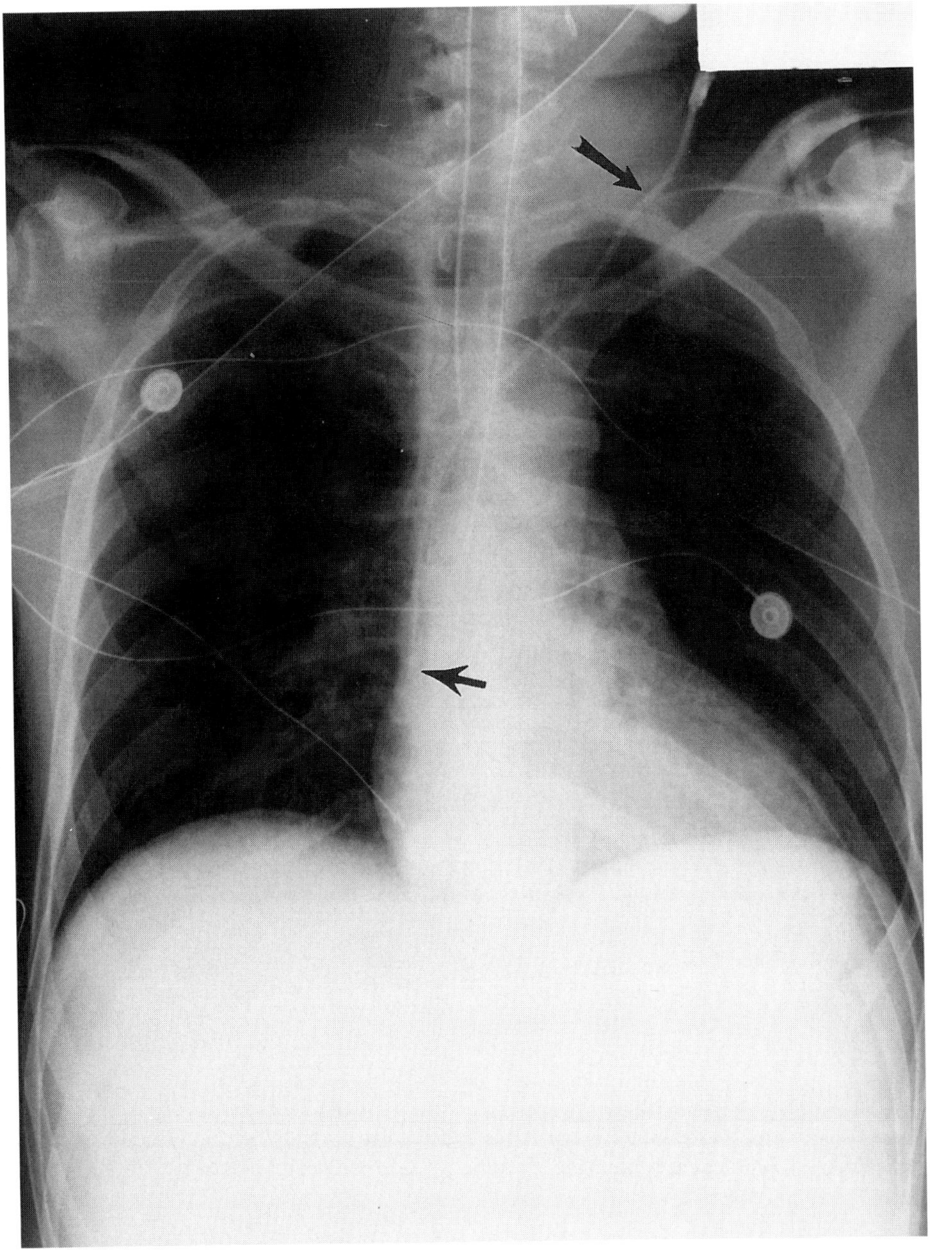

Fig. 3-4 This patient has an invasive central venous catheter in place. It enters the internal jugular vein and extends into the superior vena cava. It is easy to distinguish a jugular from a subclavian catheter because the jugular catheter follows the jawline not the clavicle. Arrows show the catheter at the jugular vein and the tip. Also notice that this patient has an endotracheal tube and a nasogastric tube in place.

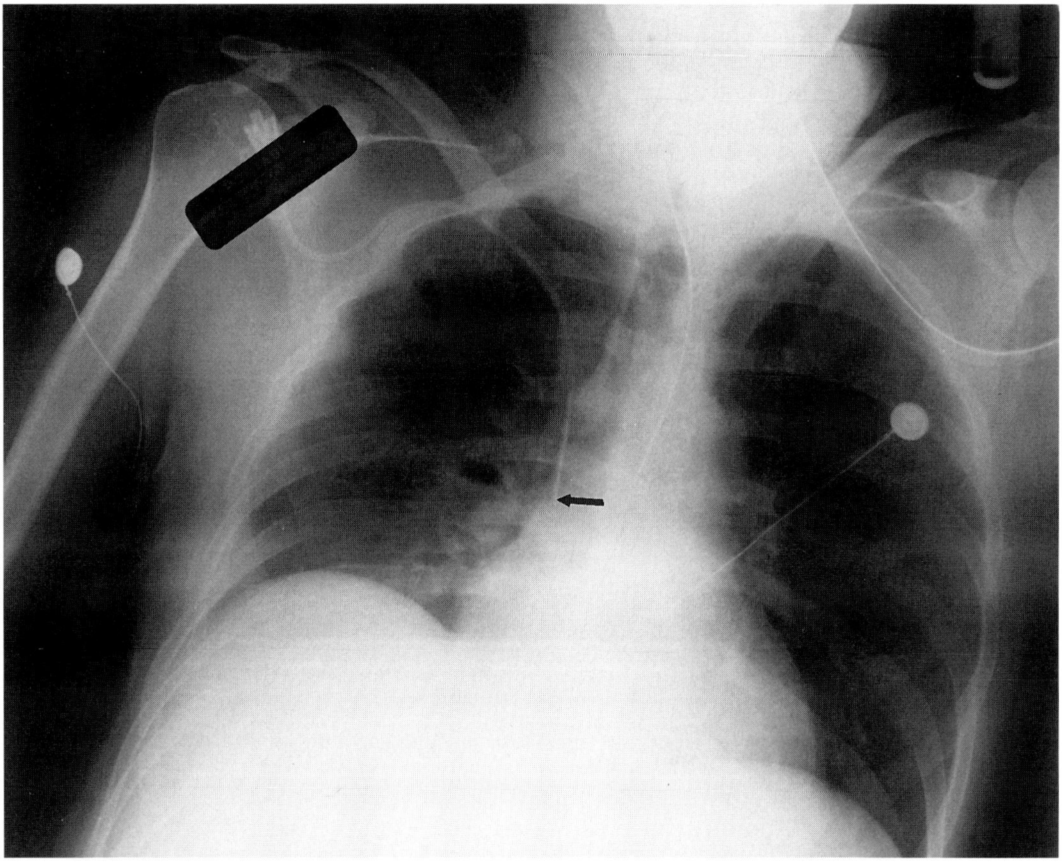

Fig. 3-5 This patient has an invasive central venous catheter placed in the subclavian vein. Notice how the catheter follows the clavicle before descending into the superior vena cava. A nasogastric tube can also be seen on the chest film.

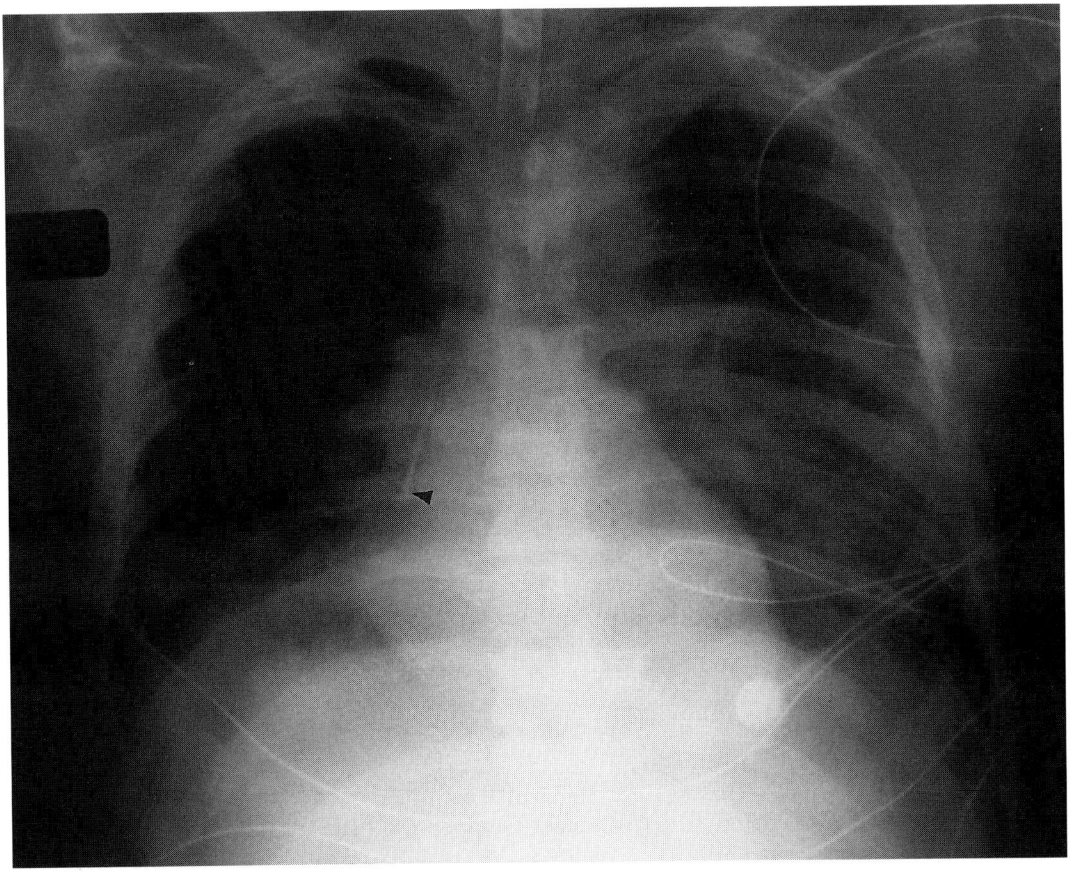

Fig. 3-6 On this chest radiograph the right subclavian catheter is inserted too far. The catheter extends past the superior vena cava and into the right atrium. Note that this patient has a tracheostomy tube in place and that there is a "ground glass" appearance in the left lung, suggesting a pleural effusion.

Radiologic Appearance

The position of the chest tube on a chest radiograph is variable, because a chest tube may be inserted anterior or posterior to the lung through an incision in the anterior chest or through an incision in the lateral chest wall. Each chest tube has a radiopaque line that extends the entire length of the chest tube, except there are breaks in the radiopaque line where there are holes in the chest tube to facilitate drainage of air and fluid. The nurse should examine the chest radiograph for correct placement of the chest tube, verifying that it is in far enough, but that it is not in too far, and that there are no kinks in the tubing to impede drainage. A chest tube should appear as a relatively straight line on the chest radiograph; the most distal or last hole of the chest tube, e.g. a break in the line, should be positioned within the rib cage (Figs. 3-7, 3-8, 3-9, and 3-10).

Nursing Implications

When a break in the line extends outside the rib cage in the subcutaneous tissue, air can enter the chest through it. The patient may develop a pneumothorax and vigorous bubbling is seen in the chest drainage bottle. If this occurs, the physician usually needs to reposition the chest tube. In the interim, the nurse may apply additional petrolatum-laden gauze to the chest tube site to prevent air from entering the pleural space through the chest tube.

TRACHEAL DEVIATION

Definition

Tracheal deviation is the displacement of the trachea to the right or to the left of its normal midline position. Tracheal deviation occurs as a result of being *pulled* by atelectasis or *pushed* by air, fluid, enlarged lymph nodes, enlarged cardiac structures, or tumor. The trachea may also be deviated in patients with rib cage abnormalities such as scoliosis, or when a large portion of lung has been removed. Removal of a portion of the lung causes similar changes to those seen in atelectasis.

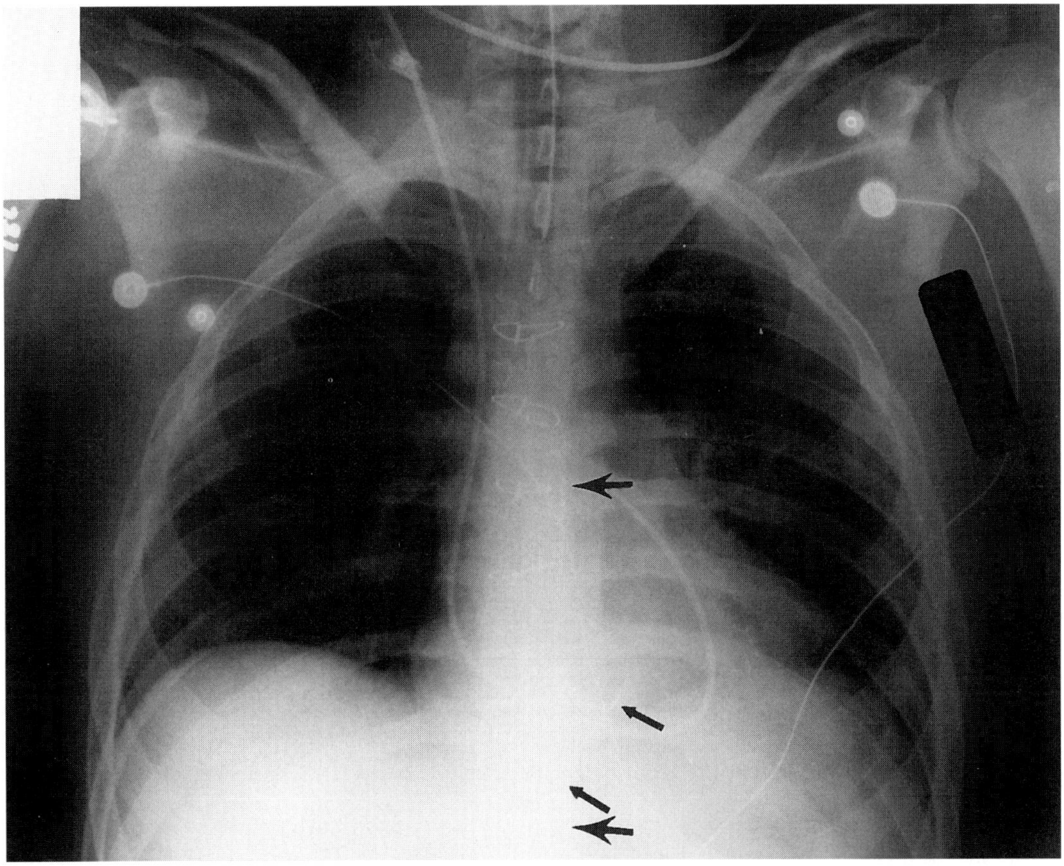

Fig. 3-7 This postoperative cardiac surgery patient has two mediastinal chest tubes in place. An arrow points to the tip of the chest tube and to the last hole on the tube. Note the placement of the pulmonary artery catheter; the endotracheal tube is positioned too high.

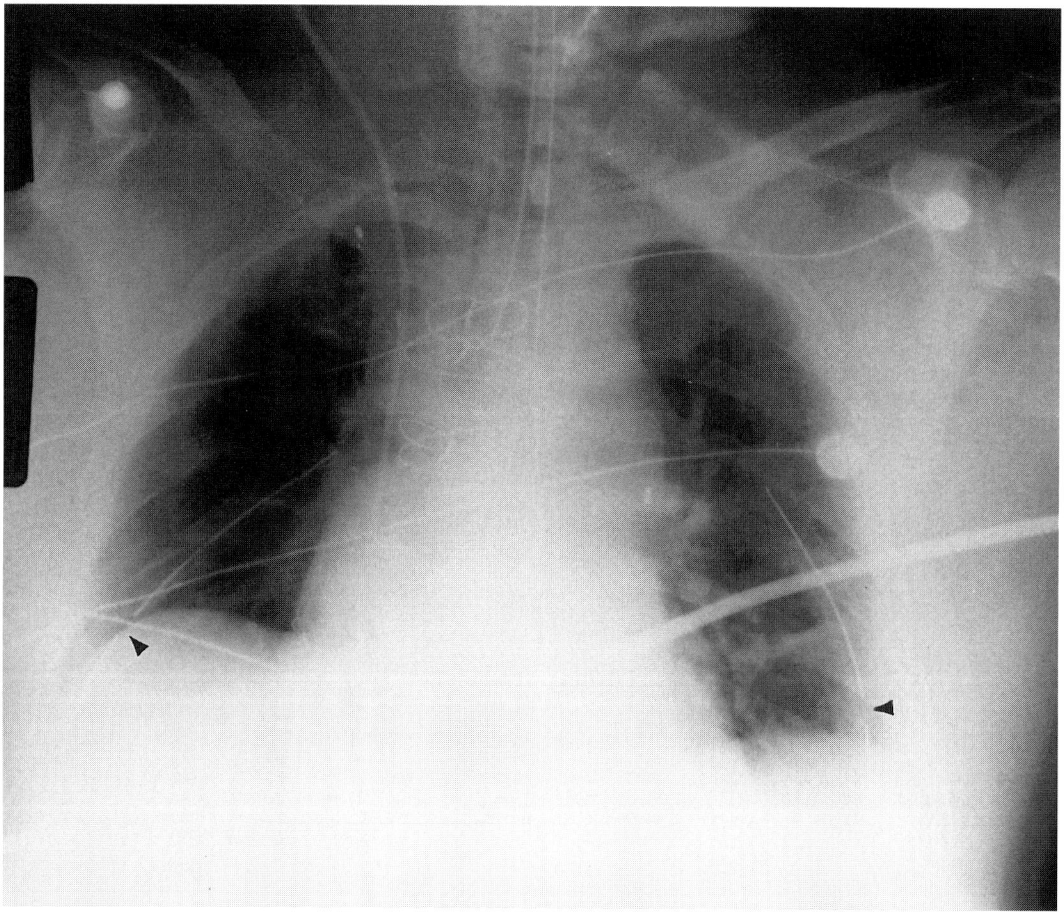

Fig. 3-8 The position of pleural chest tubes are identified on a radiograph by a thin radiopaque line, usually with a break at the position of the last hole. Notice that the last hole is in the rib cage, the tube does not extend too high in the chest, and the tube in not kinked.

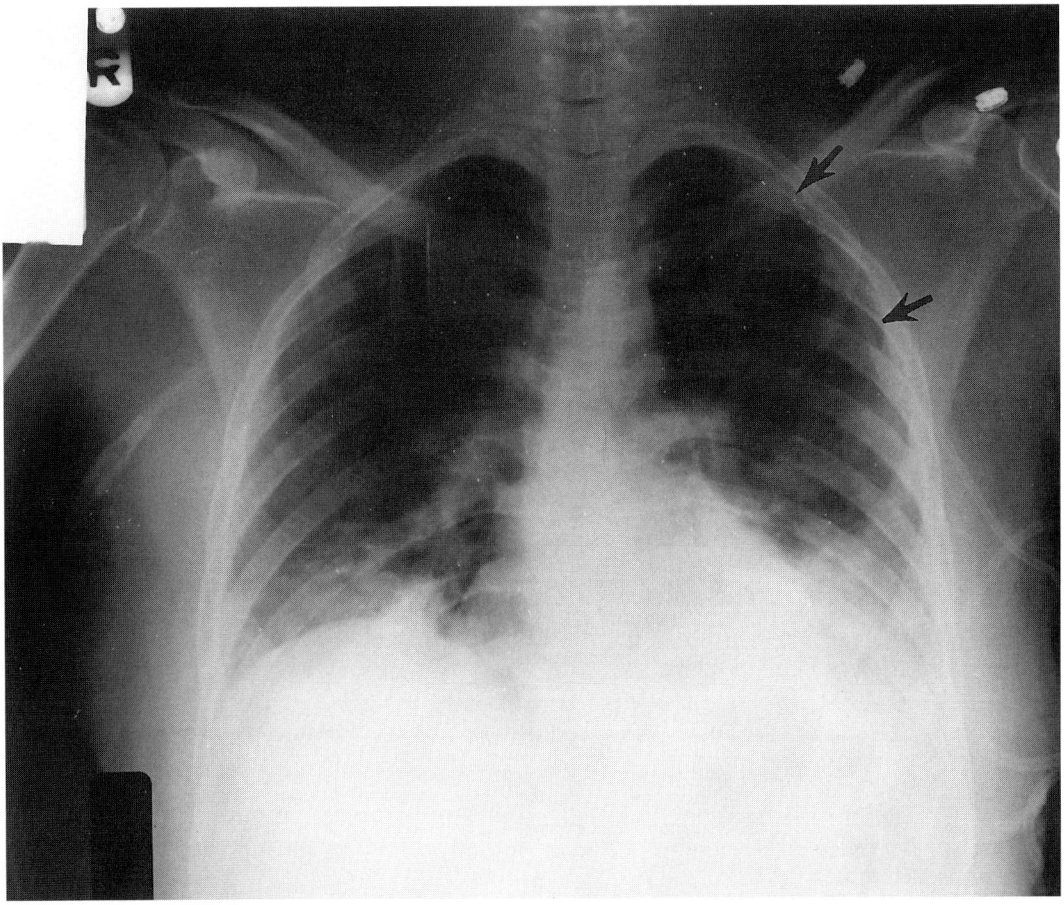

Fig. 3-9 A percutaneous pneumothorax (Cook) catheter can be seen in the upper left side of the chest. Unlike a conventional chest tube, the silhouette of a pneumothorax catheter is very thick.

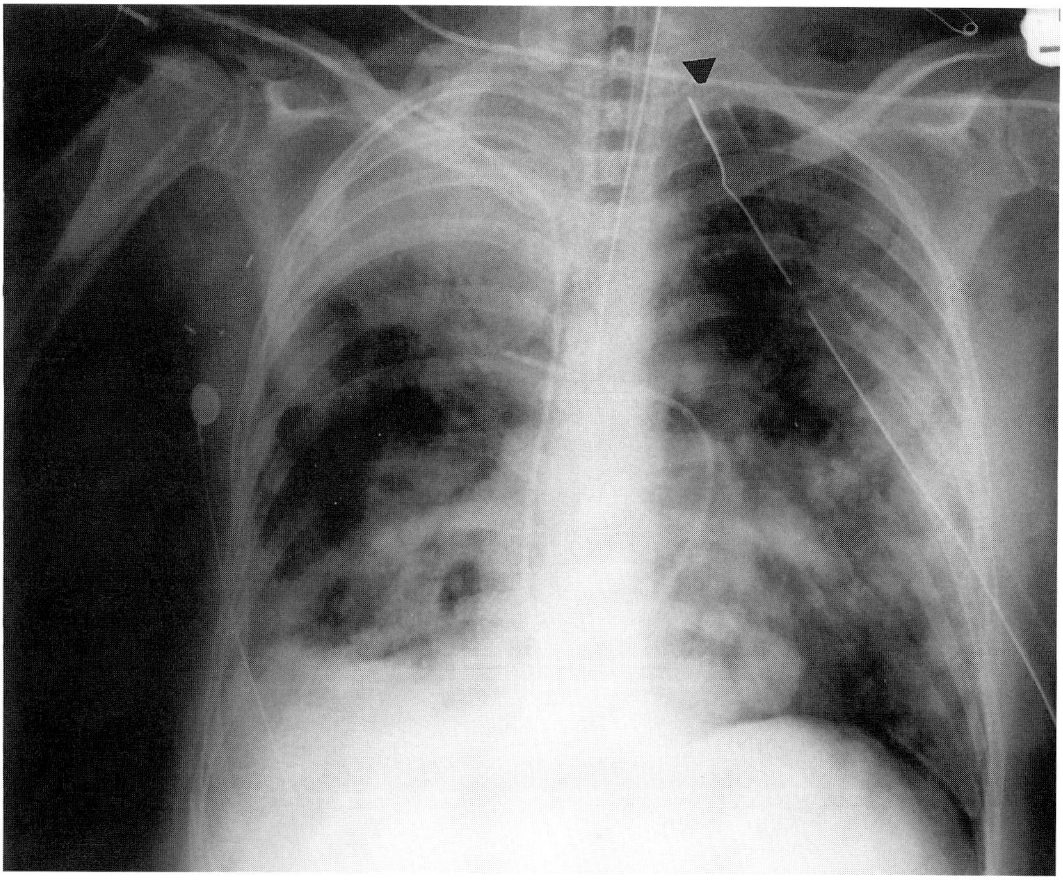

Fig. 3-10 The chest tube in the left hemithorax on this chest radiograph is inserted too far. Notice the bump in the chest tube that may impede drainage. This critically ill patient also has an endotracheal tube that is positioned too high, a left subclavian pulmonary artery catheter, and a nasogastric tube in place.

Clinical Findings

Assessment of tracheal deviation is begun by the nurse positioning the thumb and forefinger in the suprasternal notch to locate the trachea. The fingers are gently moved from left to right as the patient swallows. This determines position and mobility of the trachea. Alternately, in individuals with normal to thin neck structures, the nurse may pull down or stretch the skin laterally in the suprasternal notch area to identify position of the trachea. Other clinical findings are dependent on the cause of the deviation. (See the discussion of atelectasis, pneumothorax, and pleural effusion.)

Radiologic Appearance

On a chest radiograph, the trachea will appear deviated to one side instead of in the normal midline position. The nurse must be sure that the chest radiograph is not rotated, and should also look for atelectasis, pneumothorax, pleural effusion, or abnormal hilar structures (Fig. 3-11).

Nursing Implications

It is important to identify the cause of tracheal deviation. Additional radiographs or bronchoscopy may be necessary for diagnosis; at other times the cause is known. When tracheal deviation is present, such as from scoliosis or postoperative changes, there is no specific nursing action. At other times, tracheal deviation requires prompt nursing action to prevent serious complications. When the trachea is deviated because of pneumothorax, the physician must be immediately contacted to insert a chest tube unless the nurse is trained to insert a decompression needle or chest catheter. The patient with pneumothorax usually requires oxygen and may need intubation if cardiopulmonary arrest occurs. The nurse should anticipate a thoracentesis or chest catheter insertion when a pleural effusion is large enough to cause tracheal deviation.

RUPTURED OR PERFORATED DIAPHRAGM

Definition

Blunt or, more commonly, penetrating trauma as high as T4 tears the diaphragm. The left hemidiaphragm is involved more often because there are

A

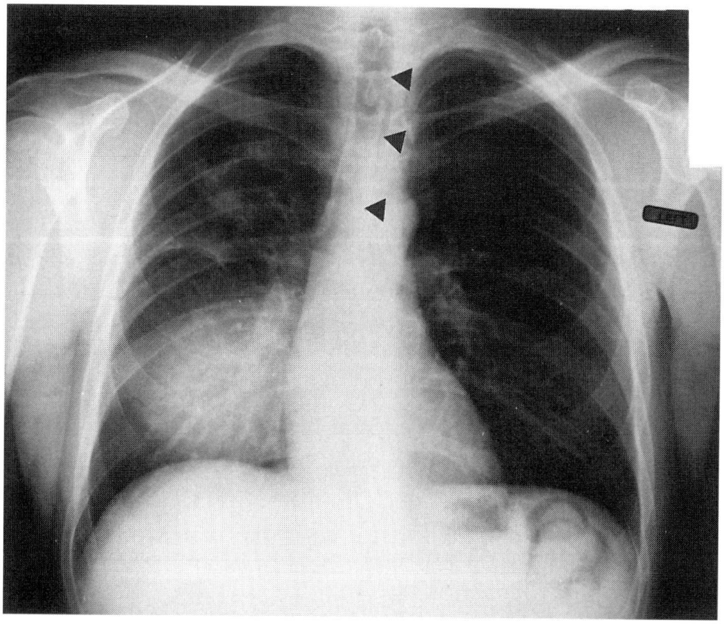

B

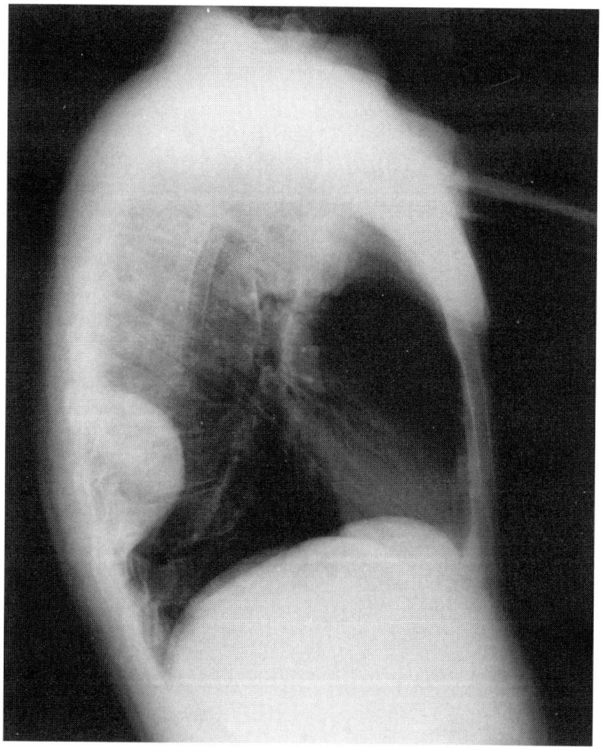

Fig. 3-11 Tracheal deviation is shown in this chest radiograph, **A. B,** The patient has a very large posterior tumor that causes the trachea to be moved to the side.

more right-handed assailants, who generally target the left side of the chest, which contains the heart. The liver, positioned on the right side of the chest, is much less targeted to trauma than the heart.

Clinical Findings

In most instances the patient will complain of chest pain in the shoulder or pain in the abdomen. The nurse may observe dyspnea, tachypnea, or a persistent air leak in the chest tube. There may be difficulty passing a nasogastric tube into the stomach, especially if bowel is herniated through the diaphragm. Respiratory or diaphragmatic excursion is decreased, especially on the side of the diaphragmatic tear. Tympany is observed to percussion if bowel is herniated into the chest. Breath sounds are usually decreased and there may be crackles in the bases.

Radiologic Appearance

A perforated diaphragm cannot be seen on a chest x-ray film, although associated findings may be assessed. In many instances the chest radiograph is initially normal or there may have been a pneumothorax for which a chest tube is inserted. Sometimes bowel is observed in the chest cavity or the affected hemidiaphragm is elevated. If a perforated diaphragm is not identified at the time of injury, inflammation will occur eventually and basilar congestion, pleural inflammation, and a markedly elevated diaphragm can develop (Fig. 3-12).

Nursing Implications

A perforated diaphragm requires surgical repair. Postoperative chest tubes and a nasogastric tube are often necessary. The patient is encouraged to deep breathe to reexpand collapsed alveoli.

ENDOTRACHEAL TUBE

Definition

An endotracheal tube is an artificial airway that is inserted for any of the following reasons: relief of airway obstruction, institution of mechanical ventilation, supplementation of inadequate oxygenation with a mask, prevention of

A

B

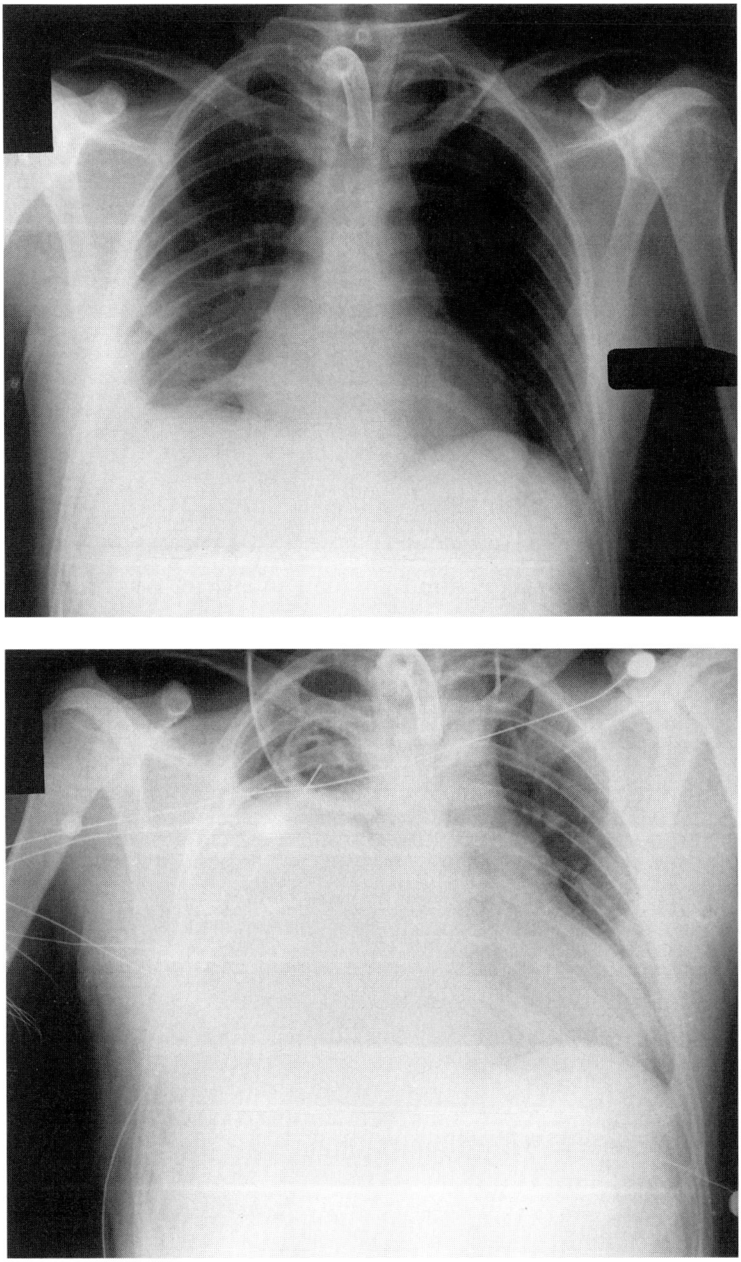

Fig. 3-12 **A** and **B,** These chest radiographs demonstrate the progression of pleural inflammation and fluid following a ruptured or perforated diaphragm. The chest radiographs were taken 1 week apart. Notice that the right side of the chest has decreasing lung volumes in site of the chest tube. Notice also that the patient has a tracheostomy tube in place.

gross aspiration, or relief of an inability to clear secretions. There are nonradiopaque number markings on the external portion of the tube and there is a radiopaque line extending the entire length of the tube. Adult endotracheal tubes contain a cuff; neonatal and some pediatric tubes do not include a cuff. Most tubes have a Murphy eye at the distal end of the tube, located just below the cuff. In an adult endotracheal tube the cuff begins approximately 1 cm above the tip of the tube and extends upward 2 to 3 cm, depending on the size and the manufacturer.

Clinical Findings

The following discussion assumes absence of unilateral lung abnormalities that would affect auscultation. When these abnormalities are present, assessment will be altered in accordance with the problem.

An endotracheal tube is correctly positioned when the nurse assesses equal bilateral breath sounds and finds that the number markings on the tube at the gumline are the same as those when the tube was placed and determined to be in good position. The patient will usually be exhaling the anticipated amount of tidal volume.

When the endotracheal tube is too high in the trachea it may be easy for incidental extubation to occur, especially if the patient has a strong cough or if the endotracheal tube is not adequately secured. The nurse may assess the leakage of air from around the cuff because the upper portion of the trachea has a larger diameter; the diameter of the trachea decreases with descent into the airways. The patient may not be exhaling the anticipated amount of tidal volume or may be making audible sounds. The nurse may also observe that the number markings on the tube at the gumline or nares are smaller than usual or that more of the tube is extending from the mouth or nose.

When the endotracheal tube is too low in the trachea it is easy for the tube to slip into a mainstem bronchus and impair ventilation to the opposite lung. The nurse may observe that the number markings on the tube at the gumline are larger than when the tube was placed and determined to be in good position. When the tube begins to enter a mainstem bronchus, the nurse will hear bilateral breath sounds because of ventilation through the Murphy eye. If the endotracheal tube is fully in a mainstem bronchus and there is no ventilation to the opposite lung through the Murphy eye, the nurse usually assesses decreased breath sounds in the nonventilated lung. Sometimes decreased breath sounds may not be heard because breath sounds are transmitted across the mediastinum. The nonventilated lung may also show changes of atelectasis. When atelectasis is pronounced, the trachea will pull toward the collapsed lung.

Radiologic Appearance

The correct position of an endotracheal tube in an adult is approximately 2 to 3 cm (or patient finger widths) above the carina, the bifurcation of the trachea into the right and left mainstem bronchi. It may be difficult to see the carina clearly because of lung abnormalities or radiograph technique. When the carina cannot be seen clearly, a second reference point to use to determine correct position of the endotracheal tube is the position of the clavicles. The clavicles are usually easy to see. If the clavicles are in their usual position at approximately the second or third ribs (the film is not lordotic), then the tip of the tube should be at approximately the level of the clavicles. Positioning the tip of the tube at the clavicles allows the tip to be above the carina and the cuff to be below the vocal cords.

When the endotracheal tube is too low in the trachea it can enter one of the mainstem bronchi. Most commonly the right mainstem is intubated, because its angle is less sharp then that of the left mainstem bronchus. The nurse may assess a "curving" of the endotracheal tube tip toward one side, usually the right. In this instance the nurse should suspect that the tube is either in or beginning to enter a mainstem bronchus, especially if there are signs of atelectasis in the opposite lung.

The position of the patient's head is important in determining the correct position of the endotracheal tube. Flexion of the head onto the chest increases the distance the tube must traverse and pulls the tube up into the trachea. Extension of the head decreases the distance the tube must travel and pushes the tube further down into the trachea. When assessing the position of the endotracheal tube, the nurse must be sure to observe the position of the patient's head. If the jaw or head is resting on the chest, or if the neck appears unusually long, caution must be used when assessing position of the endotracheal tube (Figs. 3-13, 3-14, and 3-15).

Nursing Implications

If the results of the radiograph suggest that the endotracheal tube is in the correct position the nurse must record the tube markings at the gumline or nares according to institution protocol. Most institutions record this number on the patient Kardex or nursing care plan; some institutions post this number on a card or board at the patient's bedside. If the nurse suspects a change

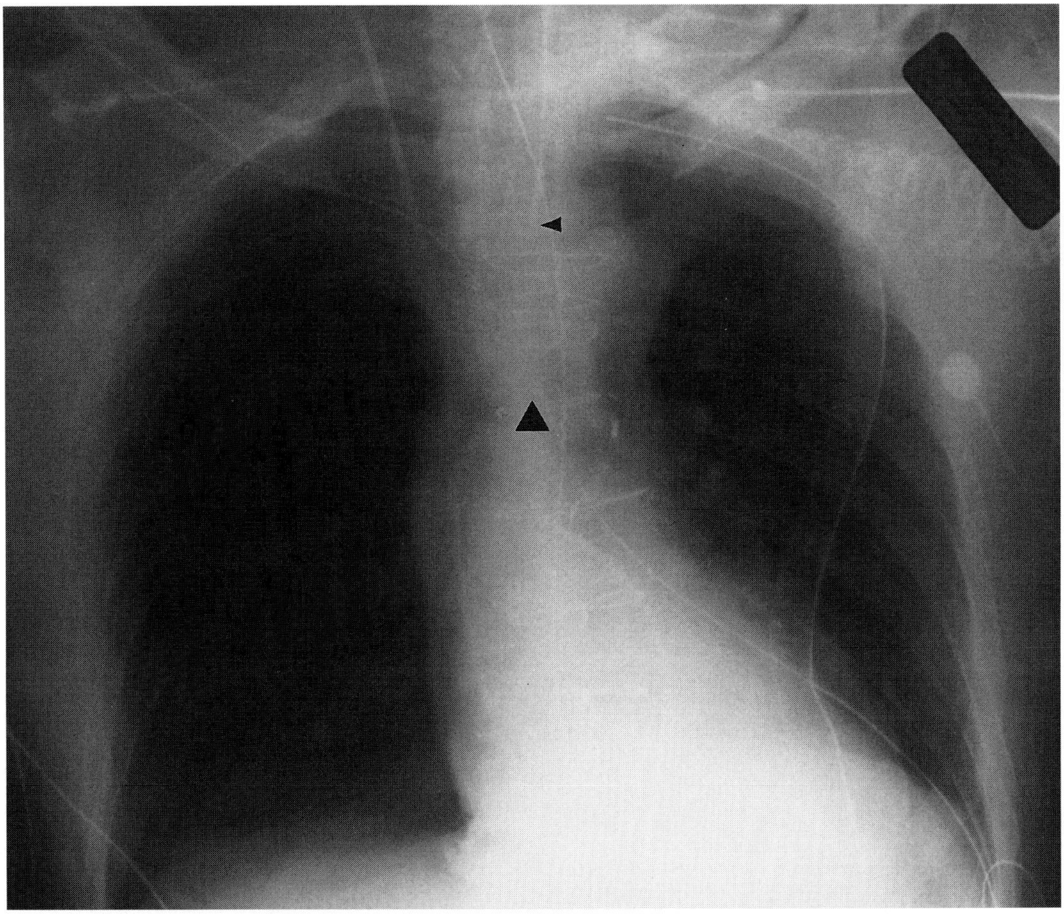

Fig. 3-13 An endotracheal tube (small arrow) is in the correct position when it is 2 to 3 patient finger breadths or centimeters above the carina as shown in this radiograph.

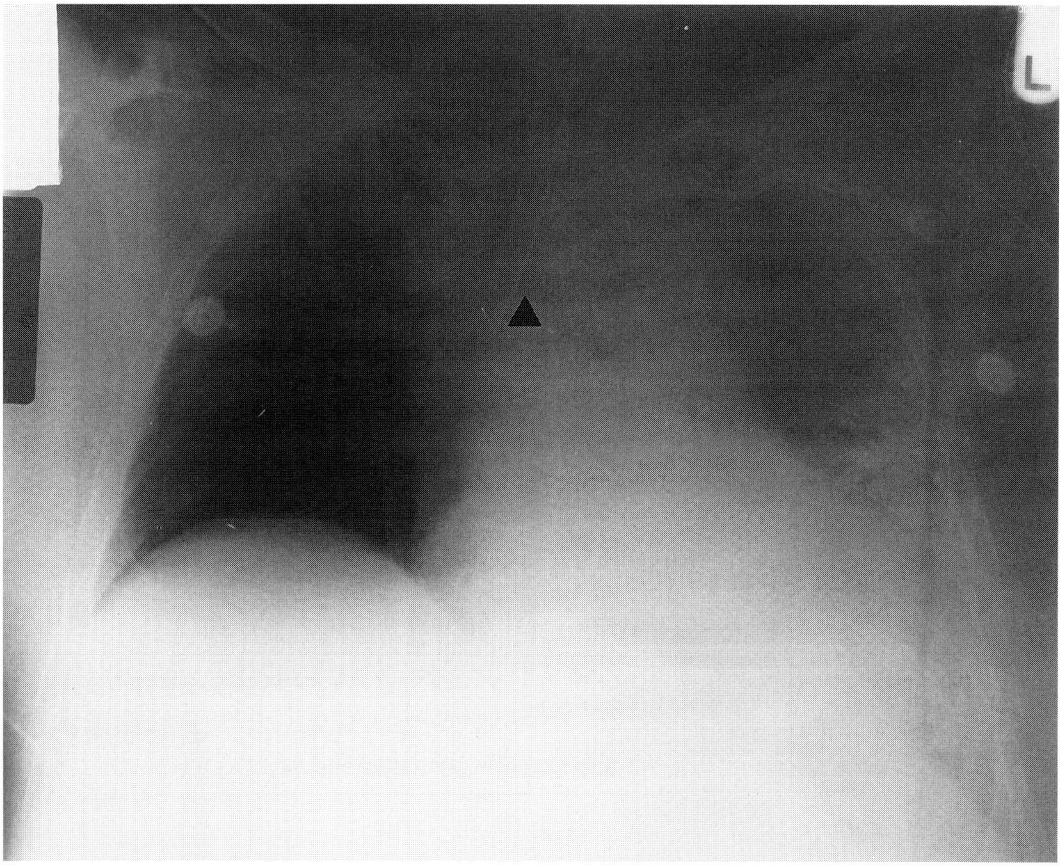

Fig. 3-14 When the endotracheal tube is inserted too far it is seen curving toward the right or left mainstem. In this radiograph the carina is marked with an arrow and the tube is entering the right mainstem bronchus.

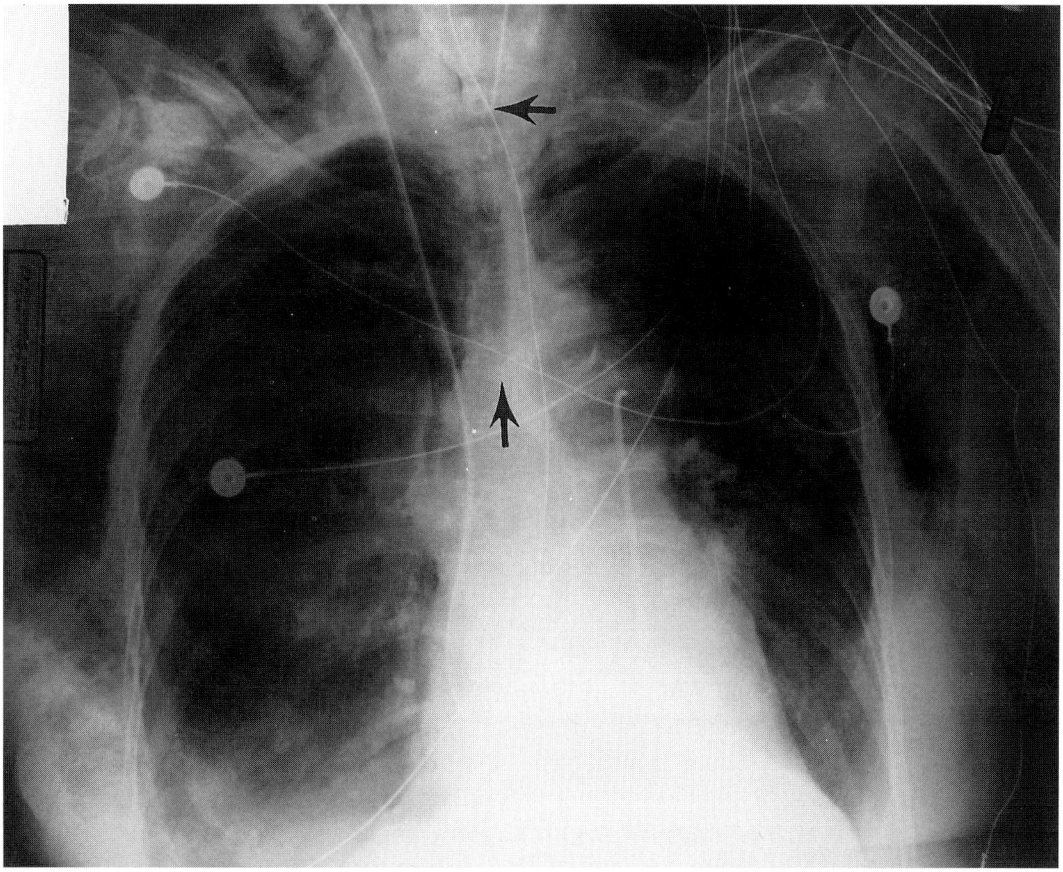

Fig. 3-15 An arrow marks the tip of the tube and the carina. Notice that the endotracheal tube is more than 2 to 3 cm above the carina, and there is risk of incidental extubation. Also notice the presence of a right internal jugular intravenous catheter extending into the pulmonary artery, a nasogastric tube, and subcutaneous air.

in the endotracheal tube position, knowledge of the correct position by number on the endotracheal tube at a body opening prevents unnecessary additional radiographs.

If the position of the endotracheal tube on the chest radiograph is either too high or too low in the trachea, the cuff is deflated and the tube is then repositioned and reinflated. How far to move the tube is determined by how many centimeters high or low the endotracheal tube is assessed to be by radiograph.

FOREIGN BODY ASPIRATION

Definition

Foreign body aspiration is common in both the pediatric and adult patient, and can be life threatening if the airway is obstructed. In adults the usual types of foreign bodies aspirated into the lower airway are partially chewed foods, especially meats and raw vegetables; in children small toys, game pieces, or large pieces of food such as hot dogs are aspirated. Nonpermanent dental work may also become dislodged and aspirated into the lower airway. Failure to remove a foreign body impairs gas exchange and can result in unconsciousness and cardiopulmonary arrest.

Clinical Findings

Multiple signs and symptoms indicate the presence of a foreign body. The patient may demonstrate the universal sign of choking—clutching the throat with the hands. The patient is generally unable to speak or to cough forcefully. There may be visible vomitus or foreign body in the mouth. The breathing pattern may be irregular, rapid, shallow, or slow; apneic periods may be observed. Often there are high-pitched inspiratory crowing noises or inspiratory or expiratory wheezing. The patient may develop cardiopulmonary arrest.

Radiologic Appearance

Metallic foreign bodies, such as nonpermanent dental work or coins, are easy to identify on a chest radiograph. The object appears bright white and, depending on its size is positioned in a mainstem bronchus. Dense plastic or glass foreign bodies may be seen, but as the density decreases, the object becomes more difficult to identify. Some foreign bodies, especially those of organic nature, are difficult to identify on a chest radiograph. Often they can be located by the presence of an infiltrate or atelectasis distal to the obstruction (Figs. 3-16 and 3-17).

Nursing Implications

Failure to remove a foreign body can result in cardiopulmonary arrest. Performing an abdominal thrust (Heimlich maneuver) often dislodges the object. Bronchoscopy or surgery may be necessary to remove the foreign body. Most patients need supplemental oxygen and emotional support.

INFILTRATES

Definition

Infiltrates are fluid-filled airways that often follow atelectasis. Infiltrates may be acute or chronic in nature. Persistent infiltrates are associated with diseases such as tuberculosis, cystic fibrosis, or bronchiectasis. Infiltrates commonly occur in pneumonia.

Clinical Findings

Although some patients with an infiltrate—especially chronic and noninfectious infiltrates—are asymptomatic, many are not. Patients with an acute infiltrate may complain of shortness of breath, fever, chills, sweats, or other constitutional symptoms of mucus retention and infection. Coughing or sputum production may be present. When present, the sputum is often abnormally colored and increased in thickness. On inspection the nurse may observe dyspnea, tachypnea, or in severe cases cyanosis. Palpation is normal or can reveal tactile fremitus when large areas of infiltrate exist and when mucus is moving through the airways. With large areas of consolidation, dullness to percussion is observed. The nurse may auscultate crackles, wheezes, or decreased breath sounds.

Radiologic Appearance

When a water density, such as the heart, is in anatomical contact with another water density, such as an infiltrate, the interface between the two areas is

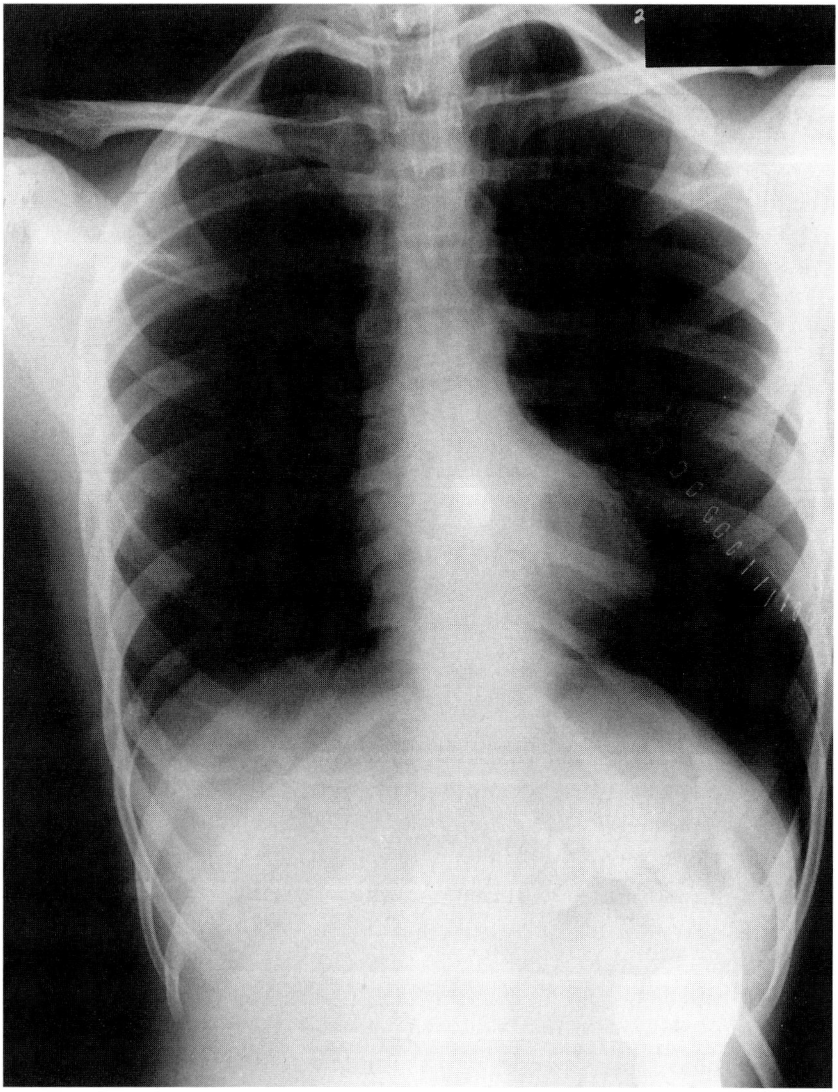

Fig. 3-16 This patient has a bullet lodged in the middle chest region. Fortunately for the patient, no internal structures were seriously injured. The bullet was posterior to the esophagus and just anterior to the spinal column.

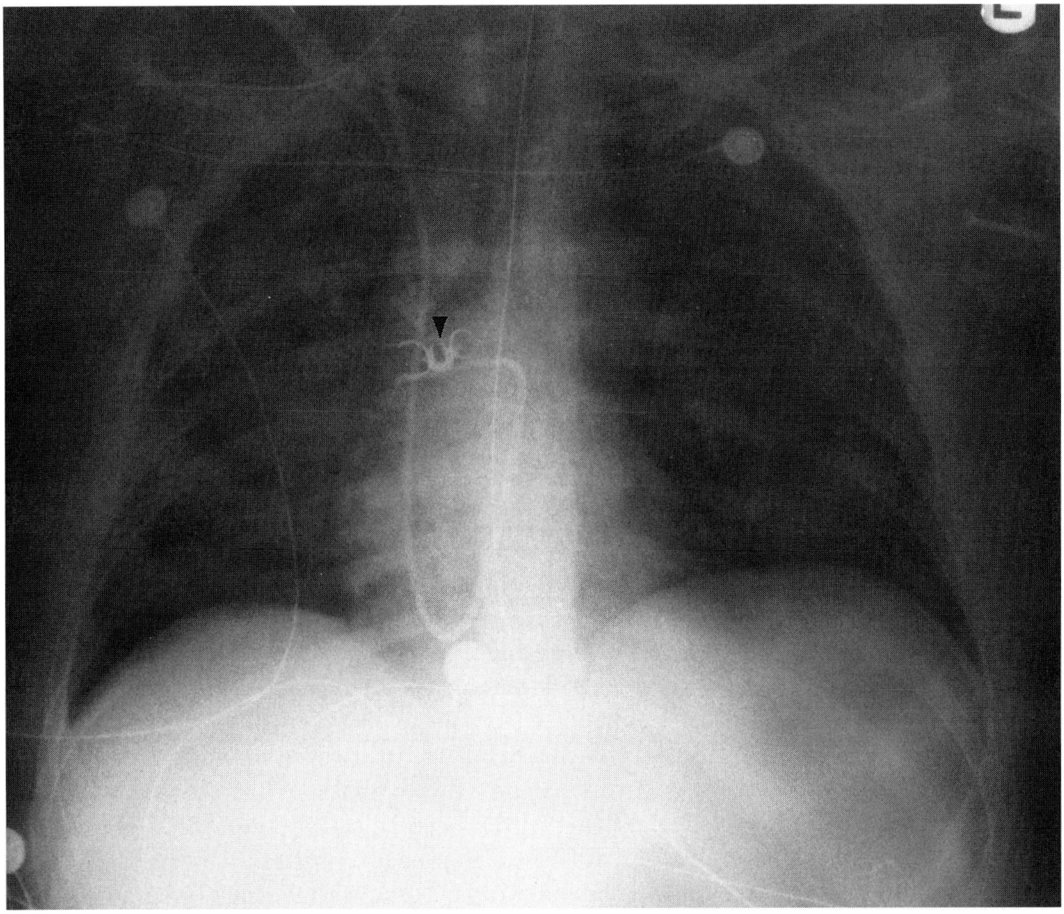

Fig. 3-17 This radiograph is an example of the seriousness of loose dental work. The patient was eating in a restaurant when his bridge was aspirated. The patient quickly developed adult respiratory distress syndrome (ARDS) as seen in the lung parenchyma. A rigid bronchoscope was used to remove the bridge, and the patient recovered in a few weeks.

obliterated. Fluid-filled airways in anatomical contact with the heart or diaphragm obliterate the border of the structure along the area of contact. Radiologists use the term *silhouette sign* to refer to the loss of the normal cardiac or diaphragmatic border.

The diaphragm, the right and left borders of the heart, and the ascending aorta are anterior structures. The right middle lobe is entirely anterior and contacts all but the uppermost portion of the right border of the heart. When the right border of the heart is obliterated, the silhouette sign indicates that the infiltrate is in the right middle lobe. The upper portion of the right border of the heart and the ascending aorta are in anatomical contact with the anterior segment of the right upper lobe. A silhouette sign involving the upper right border of the heart and the ascending aorta indicates infiltration of the anterior segment of the right upper lobe. Most of the left border of the heart is in anatomical contact with the lingula of the left upper lobe. Infiltrates in the lingula cause a silhouette sign or obliteration of the left border of the heart. The upper portion of the left border of the heart is in anatomical contact with the anterior segment of the left upper lobe. An indefinite upper left border of the heart is associated with collapse and infiltration of the anterior segment of the left upper lobe.

Posterior structures in the chest include the aortic knob, descending aorta, and left and right lower lobes. The aortic knob is the point where the ascending, transverse, and descending aortas converge in the chest. On a chest radiograph this area looks like a doorknob sticking out of the thoracic vertebrae. The apical posterior segment of the left upper lobe is in anatomical contact with the aortic knob. Disease in the apical posterior segment of the left upper lobe causes a silhouette sign of the aortic knob. The lower lobes are not in anatomical contact with the heart; infiltrates in these lobes do not cause a silhouette sign involving the heart borders. When the lower lobes of the lung are involved, the heart borders can be clearly seen through the infiltrate, unless anterior infiltrates are also present. Infiltrates in the lower lobes often cause obliteration of the diaphragm because they are in anatomical contact with the diaphragm. Infiltrates in the superior segment of the right or left lower lobes overlap the middle portion of the heart, but the heart border is not obliterated because the superior segments are posterior structures. Disease in the superior segment of the left lower lobe may also obscure the descending aorta just below the aortic knob (Fig. 3-18).

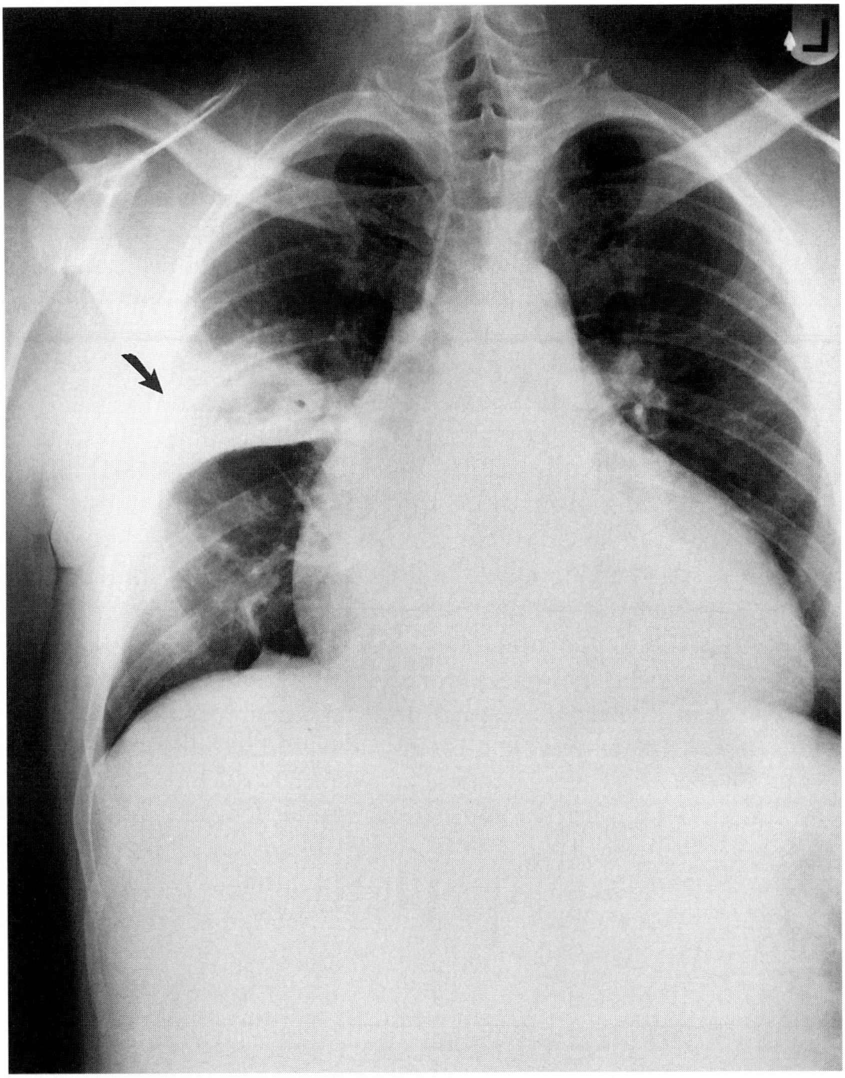

Fig. 3-18 This infiltrate is located in the right middle lung field. It is in the upper lobe because the heart border is not obliterated. Also notice that the patient has an enlarged heart.

Nursing Implications

When an infiltrate is observed, it is important to identify the cause so that treatment can be effective. The patient may need to expel mucus or undergo bronchoscopy for brushing, lavage, or biopsy specimens for laboratory examination. In patients with chronic noninfectious infiltrates there may be no specific therapy. When tumor is the cause, the patient may undergo chemotherapy, radiation, or surgery. If the infiltrate is infectious, it is important for the nurse to encourage deep breathing and coughing to reexpand the alveoli and expel the mucus. Antibiotics need to be administered as ordered by the physician. In some patients, chest physical therapy may be useful in mobilizing secretions from distal to proximal airways. The nurse should use the chest radiograph to determine effective positioning for chest physical therapy.

INTRAAORTIC BALLOON PUMP

Definition

An intraaortic balloon pump is a device that augments diastolic filling in patients with acute left ventricular cardiac failure. The catheter is usually placed through the femoral artery and threaded up into the aorta just distal to the left subclavian artery during cardiac catheterization, cardiothoracic surgery or in the ICU. At the end of the catheter is a nonporous, inflatable balloon that inflates during diastole, forcing blood into the coronary sinus.

Clinical Findings

The patient who needs an intraaortic balloon pump generally has a low cardiac output following an acute myocardial infarction or unstable angina. The patient is often hypotensive and may be cyanotic.

Radiologic Appearance

Only the tip of the balloon pump is radiopaque. On a chest radiograph the tip of the intraaortic balloon should be located just below the top of the aortic knob and at the lower border of the transverse aorta, which is just distal to the origin of the left subclavian artery. Positioning the catheter distal to this point, lower in the aorta, may cause inadequate augmentation. The tip of the intraaortic balloon pump can also migrate into the aortic arch and occlude the left subclavian artery. If the aortic balloon pump catheter is seen turning left toward the aortic valve and subclavian artery, it is in too far and must be pulled back. More proximal positioning of the balloon pump catheter increases the risk of cerebral embolization and arterial laceration (Fig. 3-19).

Nursing Implications

If the patient loses his left radial or brachial pulse, the nurse should be concerned that the balloon tip has migrated past the left subclavian artery. A chest radiograph or fluoroscopy confirms the position of the tip of the catheter. Failure to pull the catheter back to a point just distal to the left subclavian artery can result in loss of the patient's arm. Further migration of the balloon can cause stroke by impairing cerebral perfusion.

PACEMAKER

Definition

A pacer, or pacemaker, is inserted in patients who have lost the capacity for normal electrical stimulus of the heart. Some patients require insertion of an atrial pacer to assume the role of the sinus node. Others lack adequate stimulation of ventricular fibers or excitation of both atrial and ventricular fibers. A temporary pacer is inserted during acute cardiac events when pacing is needed to restore electrical impulses. If the patient demonstrates a continuing need for cardiac pacing, a permanent pacer is inserted surgically.

Clinical Findings

Prior to insertion of a pacemaker, the patient may have a variety of cardiac rhythms, including bradycardia, supraventricular tachycardia, or asystole. The patient may also have low cardiac output and cyanosis.

Radiologic Appearance

The pacemaker is inserted into the right atrial appendage or floated through the right atrium and into the right ventricle. With a temporary pacemaker, the nurse should see a "boot heel" bend as the wire passes through the right atrium and into the right ventricle. The tip of the catheter should be firmly against the ventricular wall to have adequate capture. Sometimes the wire

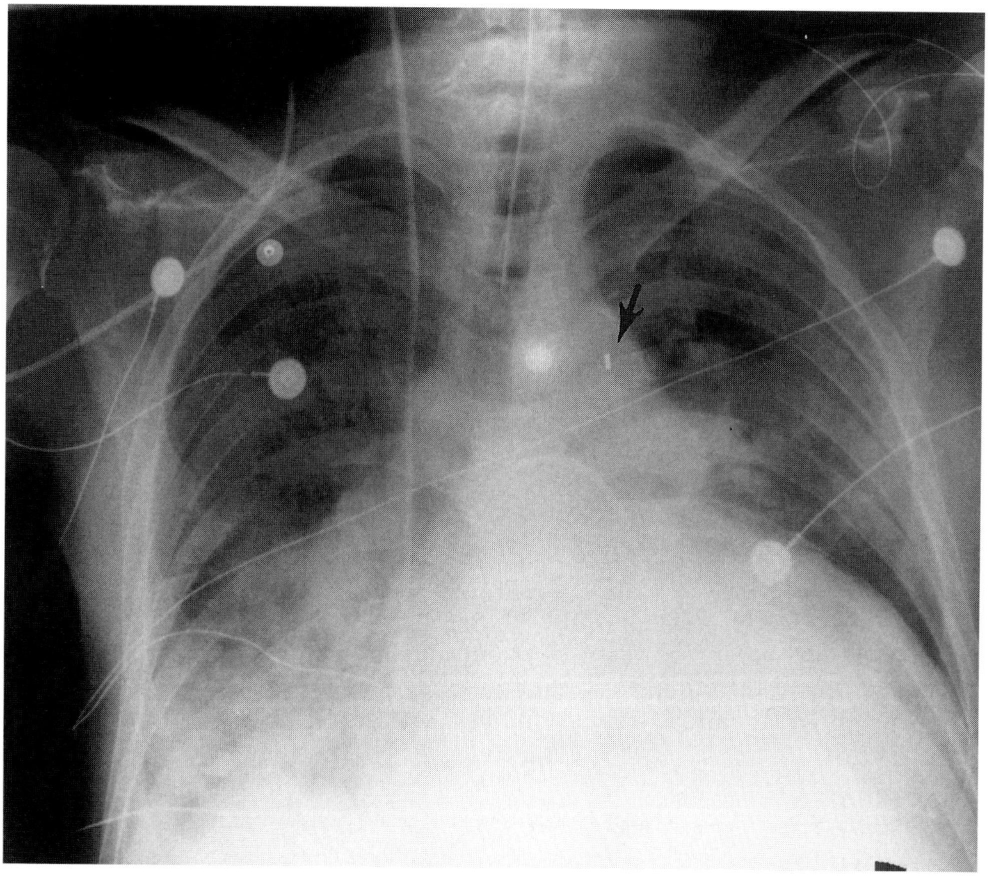

Fig. 3-19 This is an example of an intraaortic balloon pump in the correct position. Notice that the tip of the balloon pump does not extend into the transverse aorta or occlude the left subclavian artery. It is high enough in the aorta to provide adequate augmentation. This patient also has a right internal jugular intravenous catheter extending into the pulmonary artery, an endotracheal tube in the correct position, an enlarged heart, and diffuse infiltrates consistent with cardiogenic pulmonary edema.

appears to float in the ventricle, which causes poor capture of the electrical impulse. Permanent pacing wires may have a spring coil or an umbrella flange, which are sometimes visible on the chest radiograph. The tip of the wire may be seen in the atrial or ventricular area. The silastic covered wire can be traced from its origin to the pacemaker box, which may be visible on the chest radiograph or on the abdominal flat plate (Figs. 3-20 and 3-21).

Nursing Implications

If the temporary pacemaker wire does not make a "boot heel," the patient may have problems with capturing or ventricular ectopy. The nurse should carefully examine the permanent pacemaker wire on the chest radiograph for fraying, which can cause inadequate capture or sense muscular contractions of the arm. Also, there should be no breaks in the wire. If the nurse observes any of these problems, the physician should be contacted.

PLEURAL EFFUSION

Definition

Pleural effusion is a fluid collection in the pleural space below the lung and above the diaphragm. The most common causes of pleural effusion are infection, trauma, postoperative cardiac artery bypass, and congestive heart failure. The term *hemothorax* is used when the fluid is blood; *chylothorax* is used when lymphatic fluid or chyle is present. Infected or pus-containing pleural fluid is called an *empyema*. A loculated pleural effusion is encapsulated by pleural adhesion and is not free-flowing and localized to a particular area. A transudative pleural effusion is usually the result of excessive fluid states (increased hydrostatic pressure or decreased colloid osmotic pressure). An exudative pleural effusion is usually caused by infection and malignancy (inflammation).

Clinical Findings

Clinical findings depend on the size of the pleural effusion. With small pleural effusions, the patient may be asymptomatic and the findings obscure. As the size of the pleural effusion increases, the signs and symptoms also increase. The patient often complains of dyspnea with exertion or rest and may experience nonspecific chest pains. The nurse may observe tachypnea

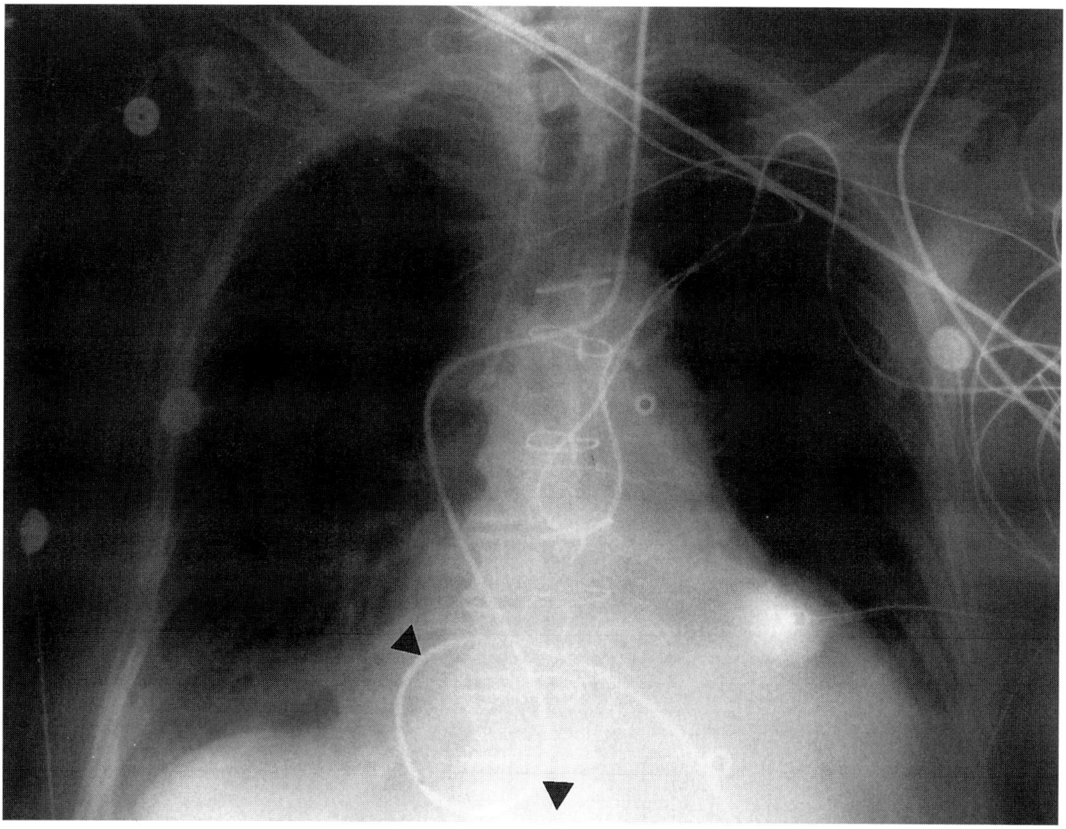

Fig. 3-20 This patient has a temporary transvenous pacemaker. Notice the curve in the pacemaker as it passes through the venous system into the right atrium, through the tricuspid valve, and into the right ventricle. The tip of the pacemaker is located near the apex of the heart.

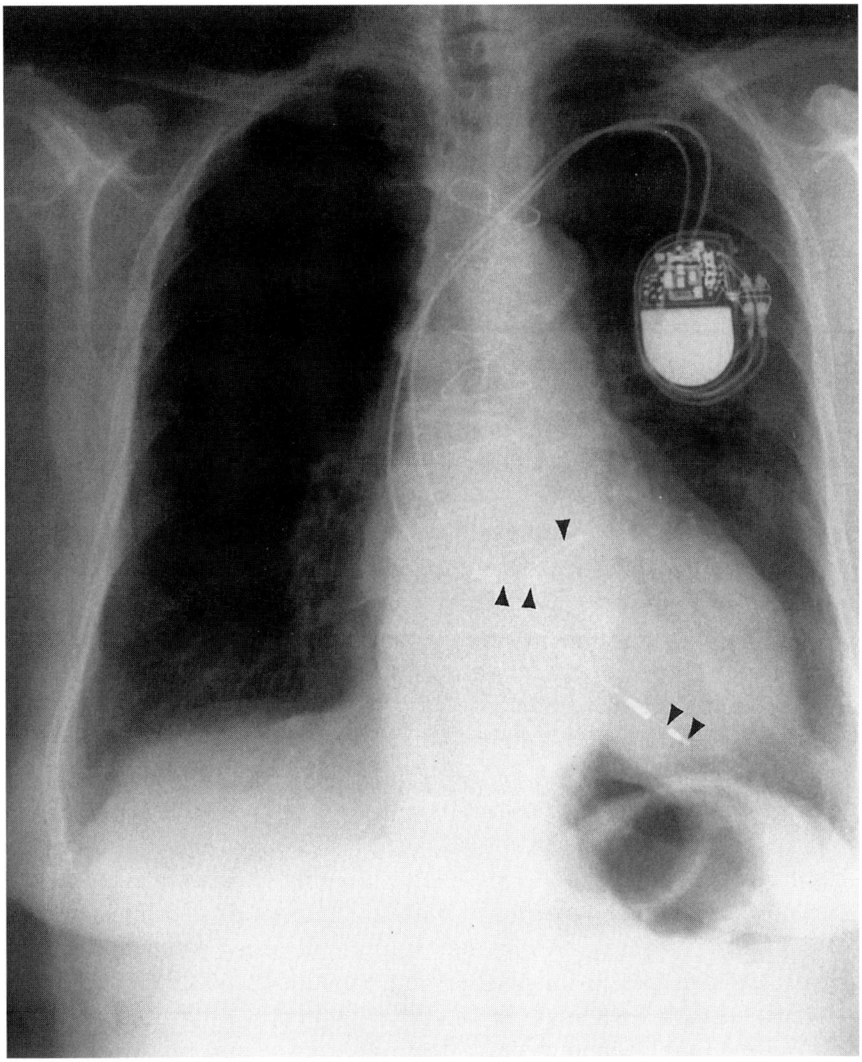

Fig. 3-21 A permanent epicardial pacemaker does not enter the heart through the right atrium. It is applied on the exterior of the heart, and wires are seen extending to the implanted pacemaker box.

and increased work of breathing. There may be decreased fremitus and decreased respiratory and diaphragmatic excursion, especially with large pleural effusions. With percussion, the nurse assesses dullness over the area of fluid accumulation. Most pleural effusions flow to dependent areas of the lung. Thus in the upright patient the dullness is assessed at the bases; in the side-lying patient the dullness is assessed in the dependent lung; it is difficult to appreciate dullness with the patient in the supine position. With auscultation, diminished breath sounds are heard in the area of the pleural effusion. Crackles caused by compression of lung parenchyma are often heard just above the effusion. Sometimes egophony and bronchial breath sounds are heard as a result of secondary atelectasis.

Radiologic Appearance

Because fluid is heavier than air, free fluid in the pleural space falls by gravity to the most dependent region of the lung. With the patient in a supine position (AP film), fluid collects posteriorly and gives the appearance of homogeneous opacification, or a "ground glass" appearance. A unilateral pleural effusion makes the unaffected lung look more radiolucent and the affected lung more radiopaque. It is often difficult to identify bilateral pleural effusions in a patient in the supine position, because the radiograph appears hazy bilaterally. With the patient in an upright position (PA or AP film), fluid gravitates to the bases of the lungs where it has several appearances. A pleural effusion is identified on a chest radiograph by the appearance of an abnormally high diaphragm, by apparent separation of the gastric air bubble from the diaphragm, or by presence of shallow or blunted costophrenic angles. Very large pleural effusions may cause mediastinal shift to the opposite side.

The costophrenic angle has four sections: anterior, posterior, medial, and lateral. Posterior costophrenic angles are only visible on a lateral chest radiograph because the dome of the diaphragm extends above them. The right or left lateral costophrenic angle is usually referenced when assessing AP or PA chest radiographs; it takes approximately 300 to 500 ml of fluid to blunt the lateral costophrenic angle in the adult. A meniscus is frequently seen at the lateral costophrenic angle and may appear to climb up (also called *tracking*) the lateral chest wall.

The physician usually orders a lateral decubitus radiograph to assess the presence of a pleural effusion and to determine if it is free-flowing or loculated. Free-flowing pleural fluid gravitates to the dependent region and forms a layer that is visible on the radiograph; a loculated effusion does not change its position regardless of the patient's position. In the critically ill patient, bilateral lateral decubitus films are often taken with portable x-ray equipment because a high-quality lateral decubitus film is difficult to obtain with a soft mattress. The nondependent costophrenic angles are assessed for clearing and the dependent lung for layering. Sometimes the mediastinum is observed also for fluid collection or fluid clearing. Loculated pleural effusions remain in their original position on a lateral decubitus radiograph and may appear to be a pneumonia, but there are no air bronchograms in a loculated pleural effusion. In congestive heart failure, loculated pleural effusions commonly occur in the fissures, and infectious causes of a loculated pleural effusion may occur anywhere in the chest (Figs. 3-22 and 3-23).

Nursing Implications

The main problem caused by a pleural effusion is ventilation-perfusion mismatching. The lung is compressed by the fluid that surrounds it. The nurse encourages the patient to take frequent deep breaths to promote lung expansion and to prevent atelectasis. Deep breathing also aids in the removal of lung mucus from compressed alveoli and helps prevent pneumonia. Positioning may be important in the patient with unilateral pleural effusion. Gas exchange is often enhanced when the less or nonaffected lung is placed down, since the dependent lung has better ventilation and perfusion.

When a pleural effusion is diagnosed on a chest radiograph, it is important to determine the cause. A thoracentesis is often performed to diagnose and differentiate a transudative from an exudative pleural effusion. After diagnosis of the cause, the physician may choose to observe or to remove the fluid. Small pleural effusions may require no treatment. Slowly accumulating pleural effusions are removed by serial thoracenteses. A large-bore chest tube is sometimes inserted to drain pleural fluid. It is important to maintain a sterile airtight dressing and closed drainage system after placement of a chest tube. Sclerosing agents such as talc or tetracycline may be used to eliminate malignant pleural effusions. This is termed *pleurodesis.*

PNEUMONIA AND ASPIRATION PNEUMONIA

Definition

Pneumonia may be primary from inhalation or aspiration of pathogenic organisms, or secondary to obstruction from a tumor or foreign body. Aspiration often causes pneumonia, an inflammatory consolidation of the

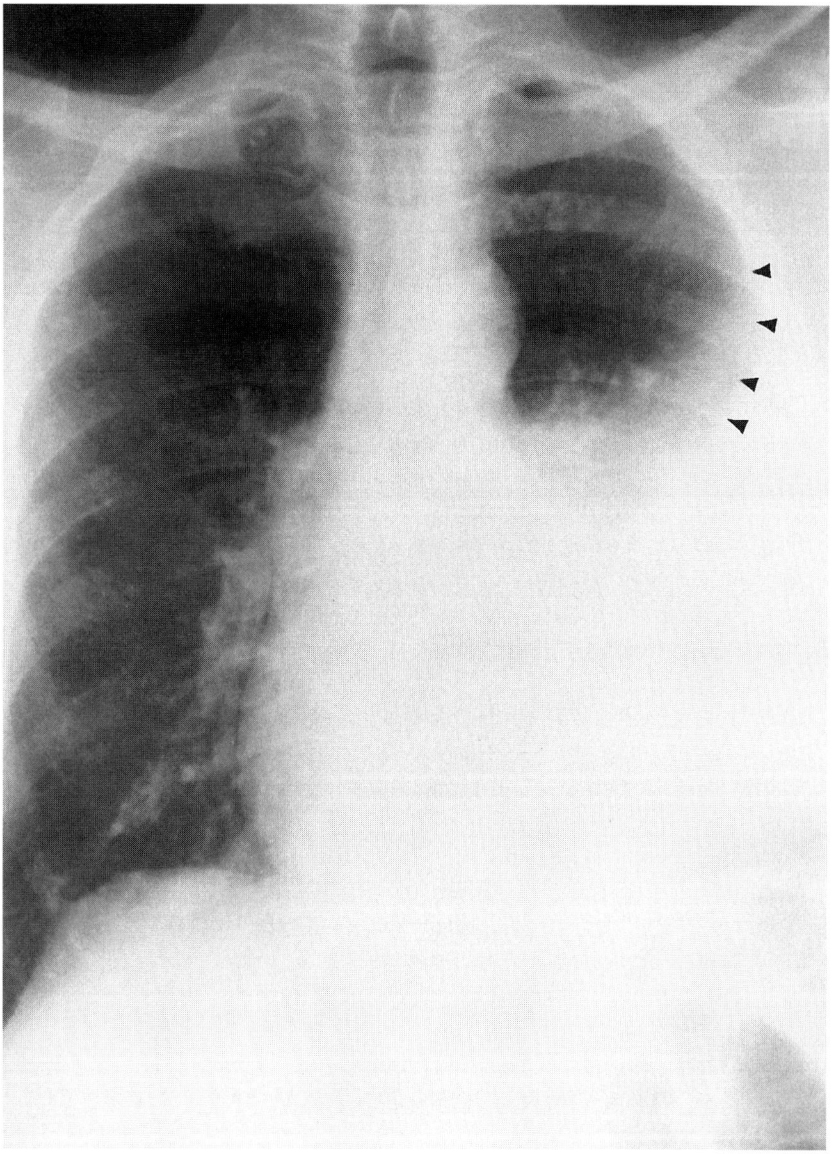

Fig. 3-22 A free-flowing pleural effusion will appear layered on a lateral decubitus radiograph. Notice the white fluid density extending the length of the lung. The depth of the fluid increases with larger pleural effusions.

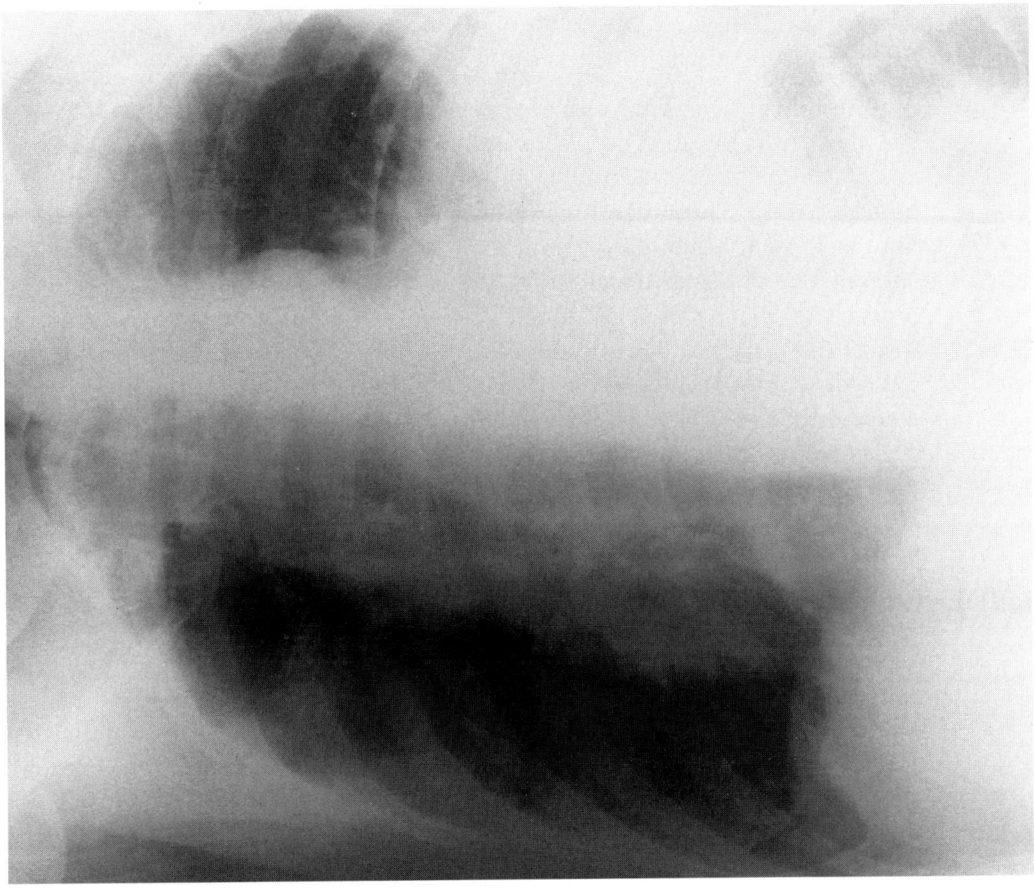

Fig. 3-23 A pleural effusion that is loculated will not change its position when the patient does as shown in this lateral chest radiograph.

lung, especially in the critically ill patient. Patients who aspirate commonly do so into the superior segment of the right lower lobe. It is difficult to aspirate into the right middle lobe, especially in adults, because of its anterior anatomical position. It is also more difficult to aspirate into the left lung because of the sharper angle of the left mainstem bronchus. Pneumonia may occur in any region of the lung.

Clinical Findings

Aspiration is often silent and diagnosed by presence of a typical infiltrate on the chest radiograph. The patient may complain of burning in the throat or chest or of having an acid taste in the mouth, especially during the night or on awakening. The nurse may observe coughing when the patient swallows liquids or food. When pneumonia is present, the patient typically has constitutional symptoms of infection including fever and diaphoresis. A cough and mucus are usually present. If the pneumonia is moderate to severe, inspection of the patient often reveals mild to severe dyspnea, some accessory muscle use, and possibly anxiety or cyanosis. Palpation and percussion demonstrate findings of consolidation, depending on the size of the pneumonia. There is usually dullness over the area of consolidation or with a concomitant pleural effusion. Auscultation can reveal normal or decreased breath sounds, crackles, wheezes, egophony, bronchophony, or whispered pectoriloquy.

Radiologic Appearance

Pneumonia appears as an alveolar or interstitial infiltrate pattern on the radiograph. Air bronchograms may be present in many types of pneumonia. Some types of pneumonia may cause necrosis of lung tissue, especially those caused by Staphylococcus, aerobic gram-negative bacteria, and anaerobes. Cavities in the lung can develop. A cavity appears as an air-filled hyperlucent area that is sometimes surrounded by a white ring. When fluid is present it settles to the bottom of the cavity, causing a fluid level to be seen on the radiograph (Figs. 3-24, 3-25, 3-26, and 3-27).

Nursing Implications

It is important to prevent aspiration and pneumonia in the critically ill patient. The nurse should position the patient, especially those patients receiving gastric tube feedings, to prevent aspiration of gastric or oral secretions. The nurse suctions the patient when needed and applies specialized

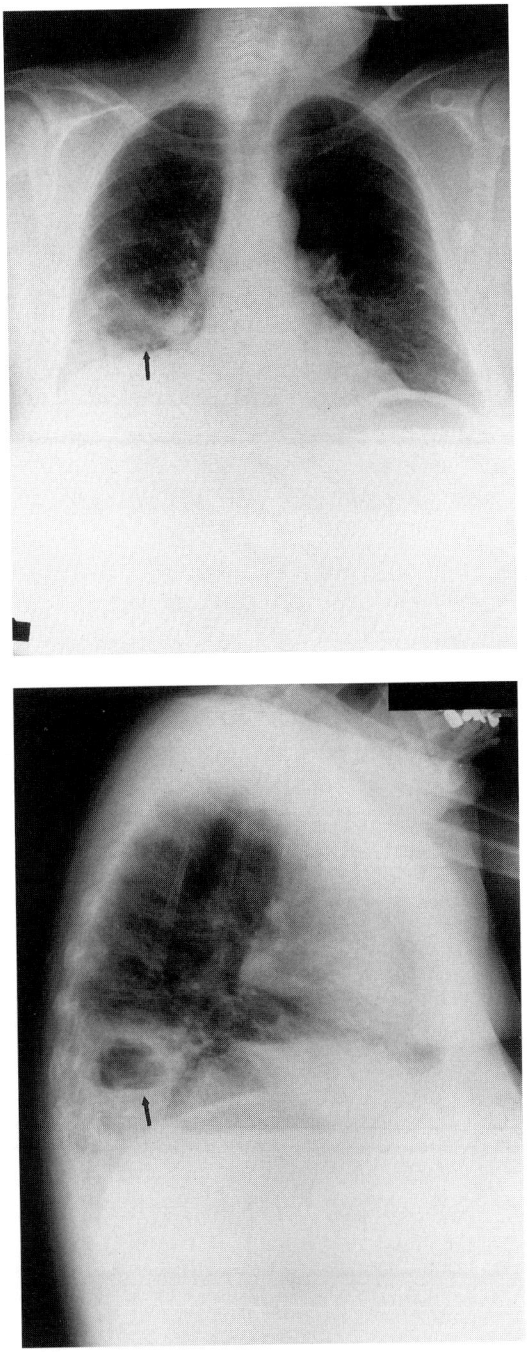

A

B

Fig. 3-24 A lung abscess with fluid level is shown in these two films. Arrows show the position of the abscess. **A,** The abscess is barely visible. **B,** The abscess is more clearly defined.

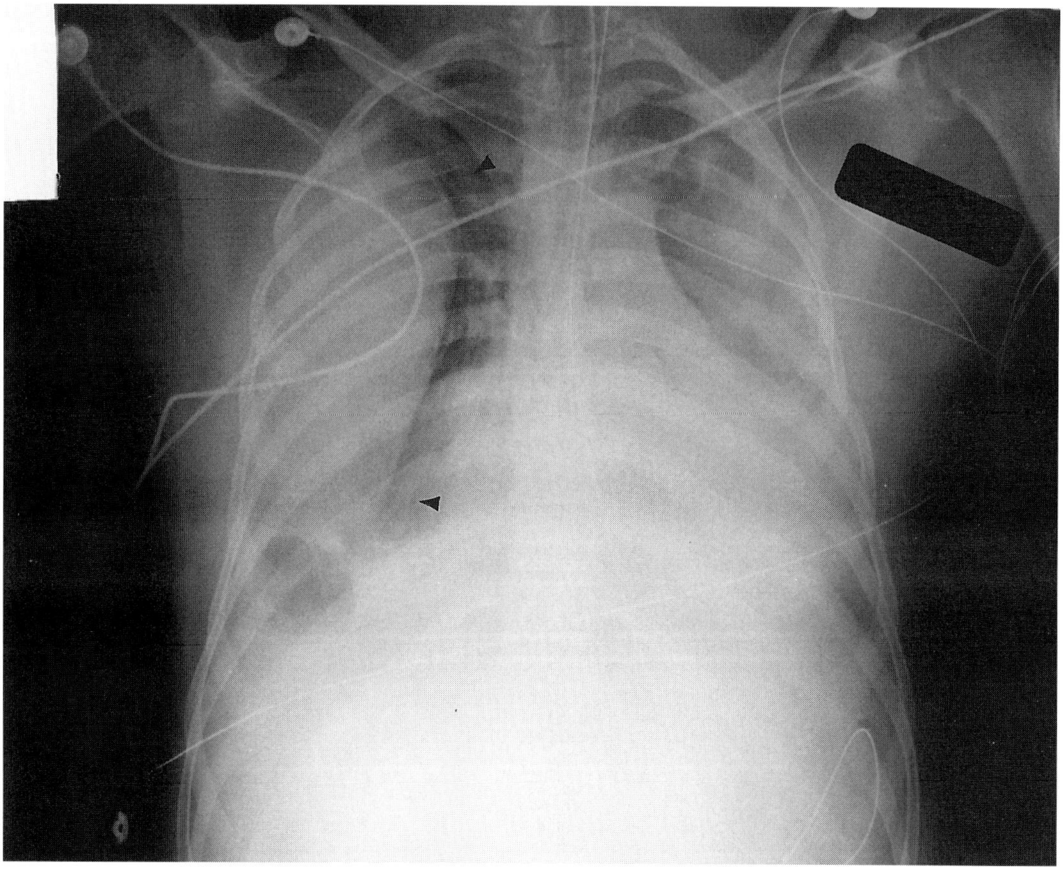

Fig. 3-25 Although they do not project well, multiple air bronchograms are present in this radiograph. The patient has right upper and lower lobe consolidation with diffuse air bronchograms. Also note the nasogastric and endotracheal tube.

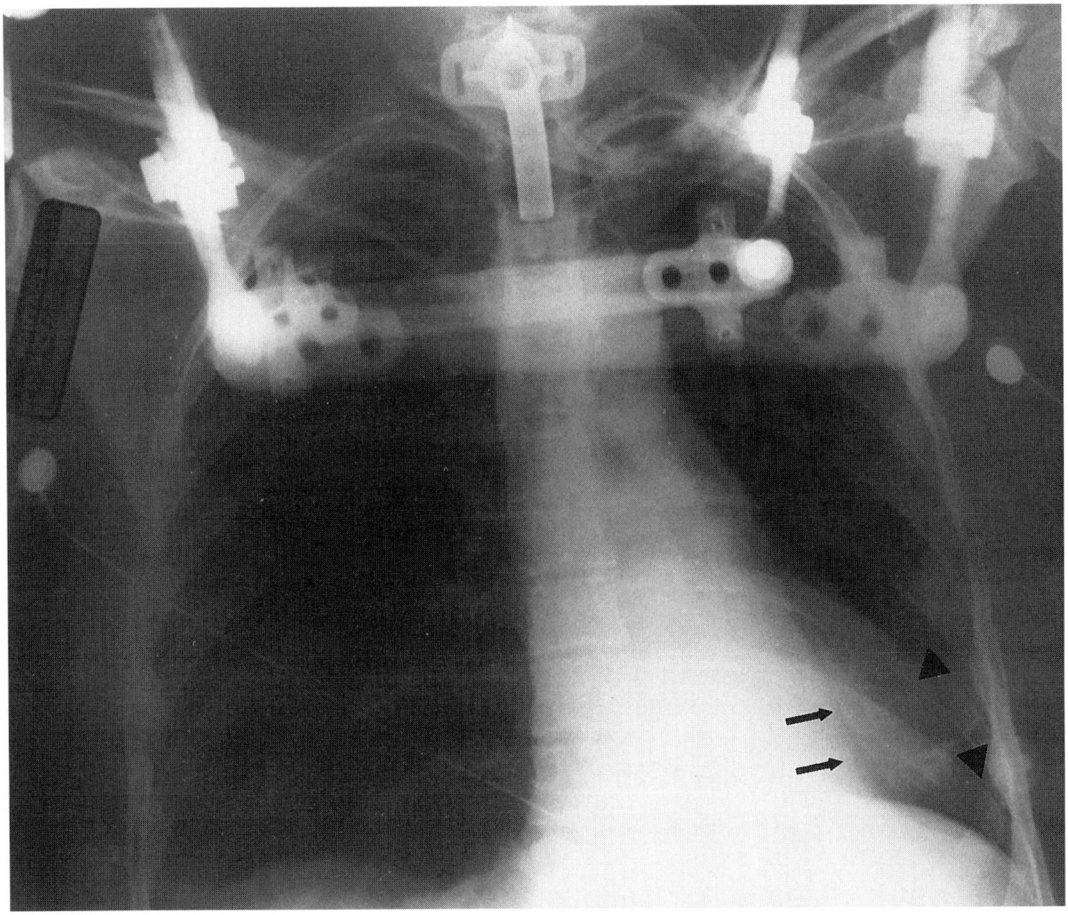

Fig. 3-26 This radiograph demonstrates isolated lower lobe collapse. (See also Fig. 3-27.)

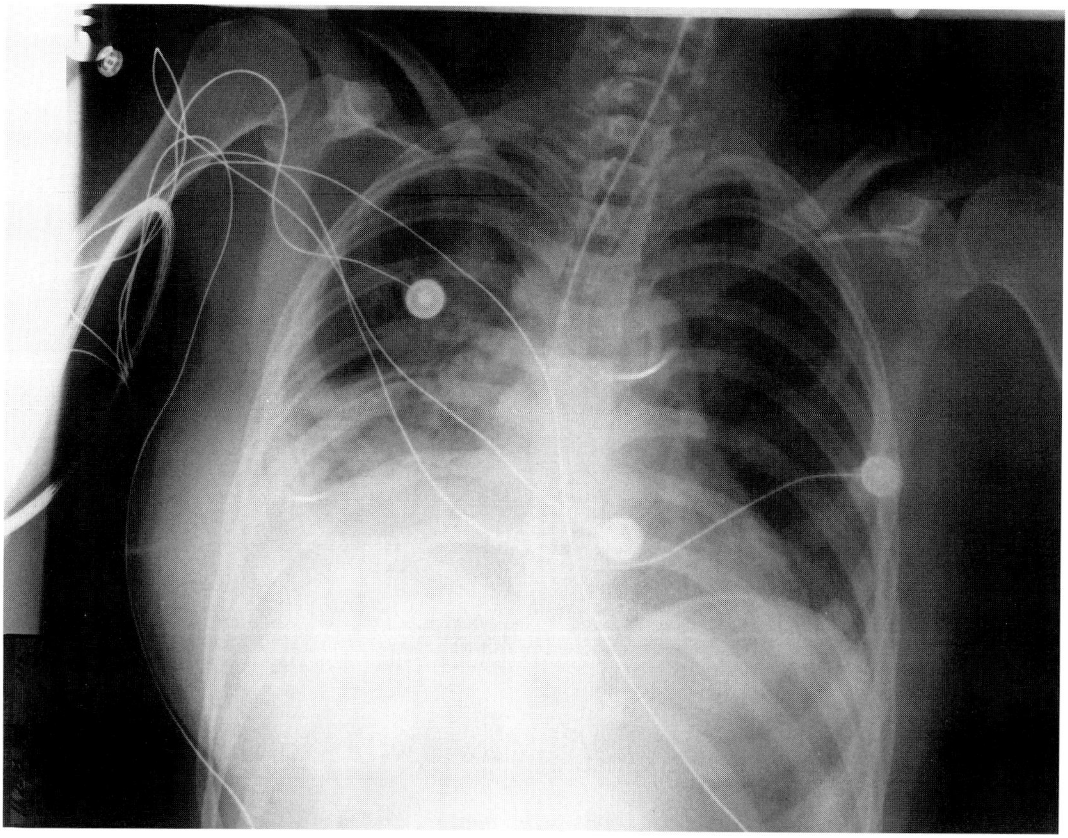

Fig. 3-27 An infiltrate that obscures the right heart border is in the middle lobe. This patient also has collapse of the right lower lobe indicated by the obscured diaphragm. The endotracheal tube is positioned incorrectly; there are calcium deposits in the aorta and on the diaphragm.

swallowing techniques with meals, drinking, and medication administration, as directed by the speech pathologist for patients with impaired swallowing. If a patient has pneumonia, the nurse should ensure adequate hydration, nutrition, and rest. Antibiotics are administered as prescribed by the physician. In some instances chest physical therapy may help mobilize secretions from distal to proximal airways so they can be coughed or suctioned out of the large airways. The nurse must use the chest radiograph to choose the most appropriate chest physical therapy position(s).

PNEUMOTHORAX

Definition

A pneumothorax is air in the thorax, or more specifically, the pleural space. A pneumothorax occurs when either the parietal or visceral pleura is torn, allowing air to enter the pleural space. A tear in the parietal pleura allows air from the atmosphere to enter the pleural space; a tear in the visceral pleura allows air from the lung to enter the pleural space. Penetrating chest trauma, pleural biopsy, and central line insertion are common causes of tears in the parietal pleura; barotrauma from mechanical ventilation, erosion by a parenchymal process, and rupture of a bleb or hyperinflated distal air space typically produce a torn visceral pleura. Sometimes a spontaneous pneumothorax is seen in teenagers during rapid growth spurts, and in young adults (usually tall, thin males in their twenties).

When air at atmospheric pressure enters the pleural space, normally a negative pressure area, the lung collapses toward the mediastinum. Perfusion and, to a greater degree, ventilation are impaired in the affected lung causing hypoxemia. As the pneumothorax enlarges, the amount of lung compression increases. An entire lung may collapse from the pressure of the pneumothorax. Sometimes the mediastinum is pushed to the opposite side, and compression of the great vessels may occur. This is termed *tension pneumothorax.*

Clinical Findings

The patient is usually in acute distress, depending on the size of the pneumothorax. Often the patient complains of sudden, sharp, or pleuritic chest pain on the affected side. The patient may also report an acute onset of dyspnea. The nurse observes tachypnea (blood gases may show acute respiratory alkalosis); the breaths are often shallow, secondary to splinting or to lung compression. The patient may be coughing, or peak ventilating pressures on the mechanical ventilator may be markedly increased. Fremitus is decreased with palpation and the nurse may assess tracheal deviation to the opposite side with a larger pneumothorax. There is often crepitus or subcutaneous emphysema (air felt under the skin) on the thorax. Percussion is usually the most revealing and specific assessment method to determine a pneumothorax, especially when the pneumothorax is large. A tympanic or hyperresonant note is elicited over the area of the pneumothorax. With auscultation the nurse hears decreased breath sounds in the affected lung. Heart sounds are normal or may be muffled. When heart tones are not heard in their usual position, the nurse should suspect mediastinal shift.

Radiologic Appearance

A pneumothorax is best seen on an expiratory film when the lungs are smaller. In an upright film the pneumothorax should be near the apices, because air rises. In a recumbent patient the pneumothorax may be seen anywhere on the radiograph but is usually observed at the outer upper region(s) of the lung(s). Sometimes the pneumothorax is more easily identified because it outlines the diaphragm or the mediastinum (pneumomediastinum).

The edges of the lung fields are assessed for lung markings extending all the way to the rib cage. Some pneumothoraces are easy to identify because there is a distinct hairline shadow. This shadow is the visceral pleura, which separates the edge of the lung from the pleural space; it appears dark black and contains no vascular lung markings. When the lung markings are not observed at the rib margins, a pneumothorax should be suspected. Sometimes the proximal margins of the scapula are thought to be the edge of a pneumothorax. The nurse should look carefully for lung markings extending past any distinct line.

When a tension pneumothorax is present, the heart, trachea, invasive lines, and other mediastinal and hilar structures are shifted from their normal positions to the opposite side. The totally collapsed lung can appear to be a white kidney-shaped object about the size of a large fist in the normal hilar area (Figs. 3-28, 3-29, and 3-30).

Nursing Implications

The treatment for a pneumothorax depends on its size. Most patients receive supplemental oxygen. A small pneumothorax (usually estimated to be 5% or less), is frequently observed for growth or absorption unless the patient's gas

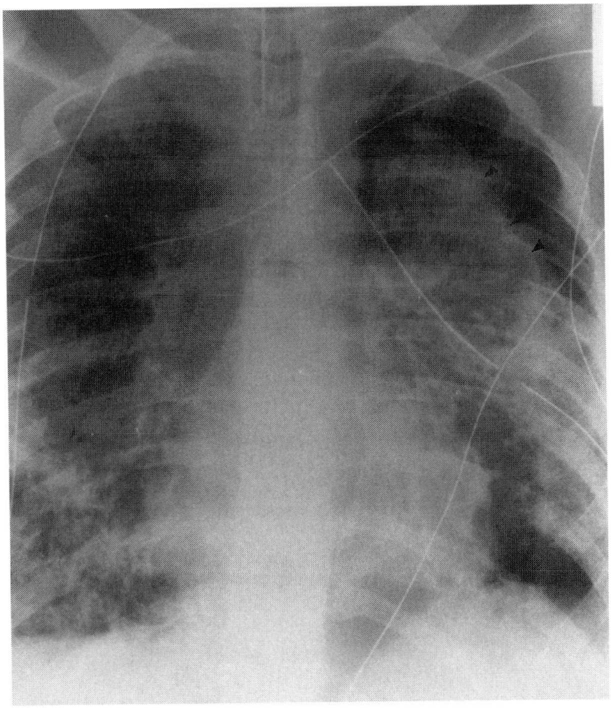

A

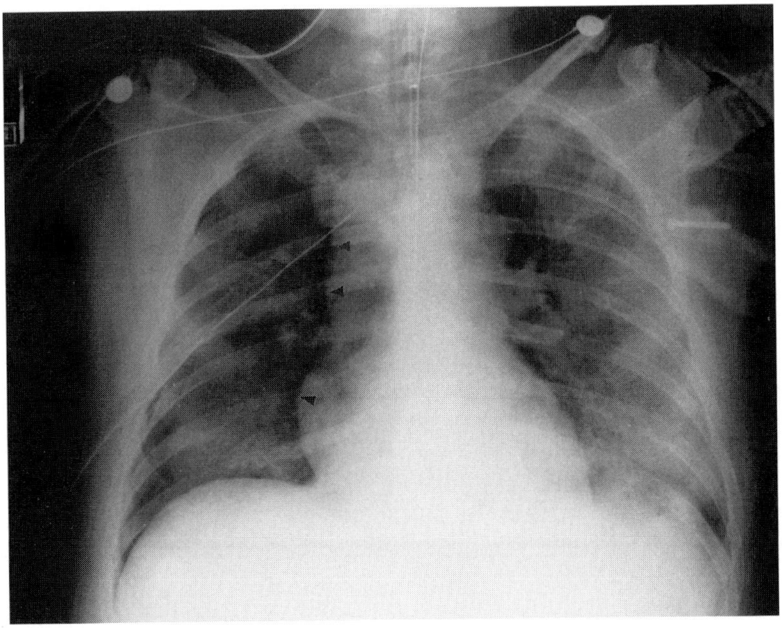

B

Fig. 3-28 **A** and **B,** Trace the lung markings out to the border of the rib cage. When the lung markings stop short of the rib cage and there is increased radiolucency in the pleural space, the patient has a pneumothorax.

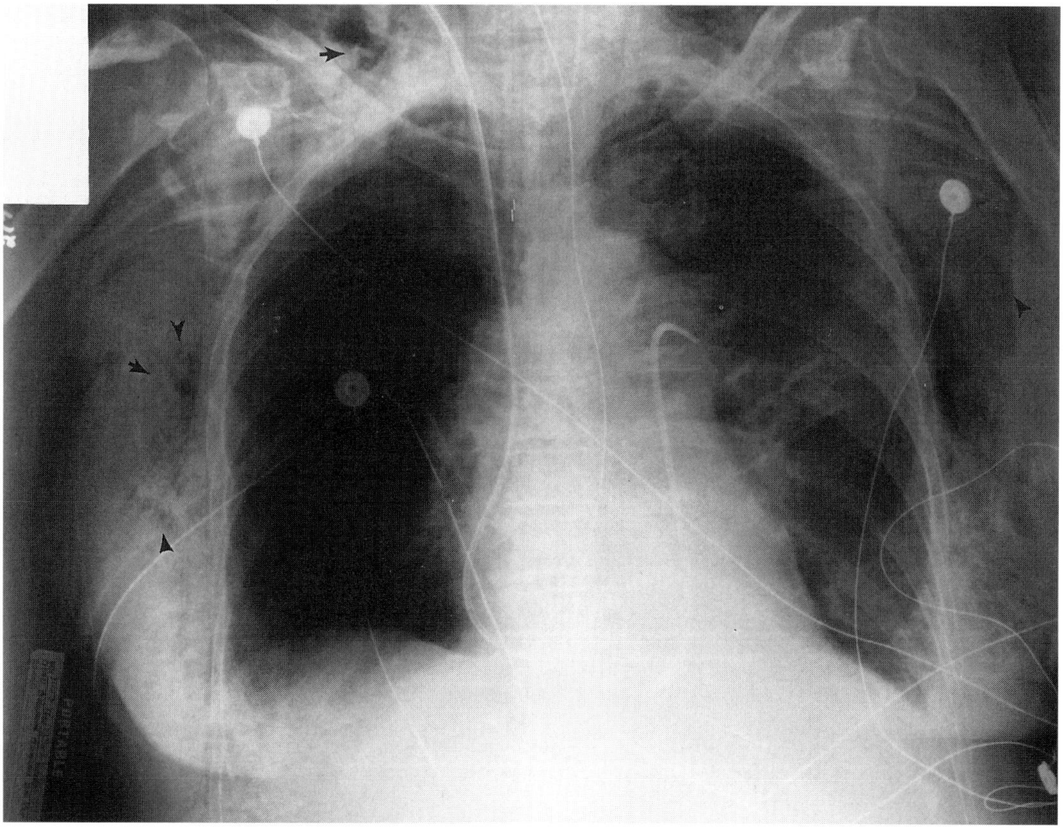

Fig. 3-29 This patient has subcutaneous air in the fatty tissue just outside the rib cage. A kinked chest tube in the right side of the chest, a right internal jugular catheter extending into the pulmonary artery, and a nasogastric tube can also be seen.

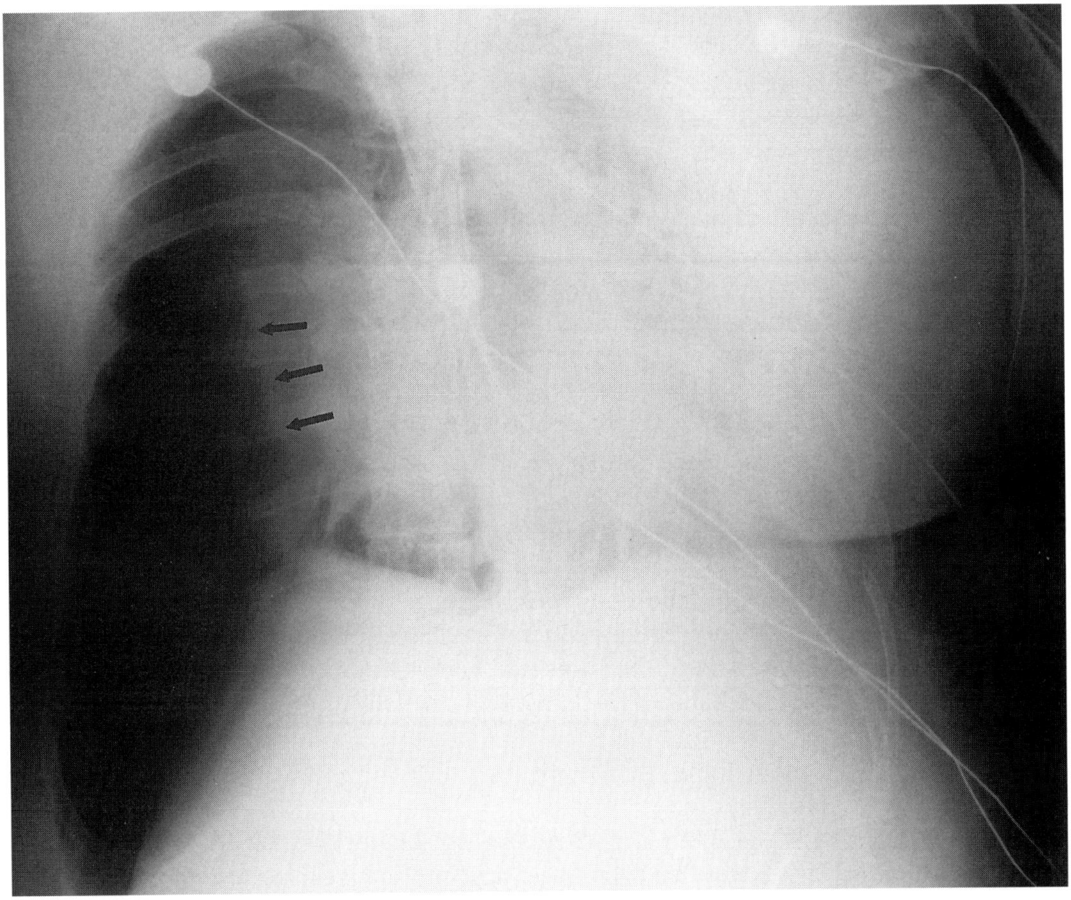

Fig. 3-30 This patient has mediastinal shift illustrated by the uncommon position of the pulmonary artery catheter and increased radiolucency in the right side of the chest. Arrows mark the lung border in this tension pneumothorax. Also visible are a left internal jugular catheter and an endotracheal tube.

exchange is compromised or the patient is receiving positive pressure mechanical ventilation. Larger pneumothoraces require insertion of a small-bore catheter or tube for removal. A small-bore chest tube by way of a trocar, a pneumothorax catheter with a Heimlich valve, or a large-bore chest tube may be inserted to remove air from the pleural space. In an emergency, such as a tension pneumothorax, which is life threatening, an 18-gauge needle is inserted in the second or third intercostal space to release air. If possible, before insertion or afterward, the needle is attached to a syringe that contains a few milliliters of sterile water or saline to act as a water seal, and the plunger is removed to allow free air evacuation. The needle or water seal syringe is left in place until a chest tube can be inserted. When there are recurrent spontaneous pneumothoraces, pleurodesis with talc or tetracycline may be necessary.

PULMONARY ARTERY CATHETER

Definition

A pulmonary artery catheter is inserted percutaneously from the subclavian, internal jugular, or femoral vein to determine cardiac function. The catheter is floated through the right atrium, tricuspid valve, right ventricle, pulmonic valve, and out into the pulmonary artery, where the tip of the catheter is positioned to allow wedging when a small balloon on the tip is inflated. The catheter allows the nurse to assess hemodynamics, including pressures on the right and left sides of the heart and cardiac output.

Clinical Findings

Patients who need a pulmonary artery catheter include those patients who have problems with fluid balance, oxygenation, respiratory and cardiac failure, sepsis, and shock.

Radiologic Appearance

When the pulmonary artery catheter is inserted through the internal jugular or subclavian vein, the nurse assesses the chest radiograph for a pneumothorax. The nurse follows the catheter from its insertion point through the heart and into the pulmonary artery. The nurse may observe catheter coiling in the right atrium or ventricle, which increases the risk of ectopic foci. Usually the tip of the catheter enters the right pulmonary artery, forming a circular loop appearance. If the catheter enters the left pulmonary artery, it may appear to double back on itself. If this occurs, catheter position may be better seen on an oblique or lateral chest x-ray film. When correctly positioned, a pulmonary artery catheter does not extend past the inner (medial) one third of the lung diameter (Fig. 3-31).

Nursing Implications

A catheter that extends further out into the lung places the patient at risk for pulmonary infarction. Usually the nurse will see either a continuous or intermittent wedged catheter wave form on the monitor. A catheter that is not inserted into the pulmonary artery or is positioned in the outflow tract places the patient at risk for ectopic foci and valve damage. In this case the nurse will have a continuous or intermittent right ventricular wave form on the monitor.

CARDIOGENIC PULMONARY EDEMA

Definition

Pulmonary edema is an abnormal collection of fluid in the extravascular spaces and tissues of the lungs. Cardiogenic pulmonary edema is the result of left ventricular heart failure or pulmonary venous hypertension. Pulmonary edema is caused by an increase in hydrostatic pressure (Starling's law). The ventricle is unable to pump blood efficiently from the heart, causing fluid to back up into the lungs and impairing oxygen delivery to the tissues.

Clinical Findings

The patient usually complains of dyspnea, orthopnea, and paroxysmal nocturnal dyspnea; he or she may also complain of chest pain if a myocardial infarction is the cause. The patient may have a dry, hacking cough early in the edema that progresses to pink frothy sputum as the pulmonary edema develops. On inspection the nurse notes tachypnea and shallow respirations. Fremitus may be noted with palpation, especially in the bases of an upright patient. Percussion usually reveals dullness in dependent regions of the lungs secondary to fluid accumulation. The nurse assesses crackles in the dependent regions of the lungs; the position of these crackles changes as the patient's

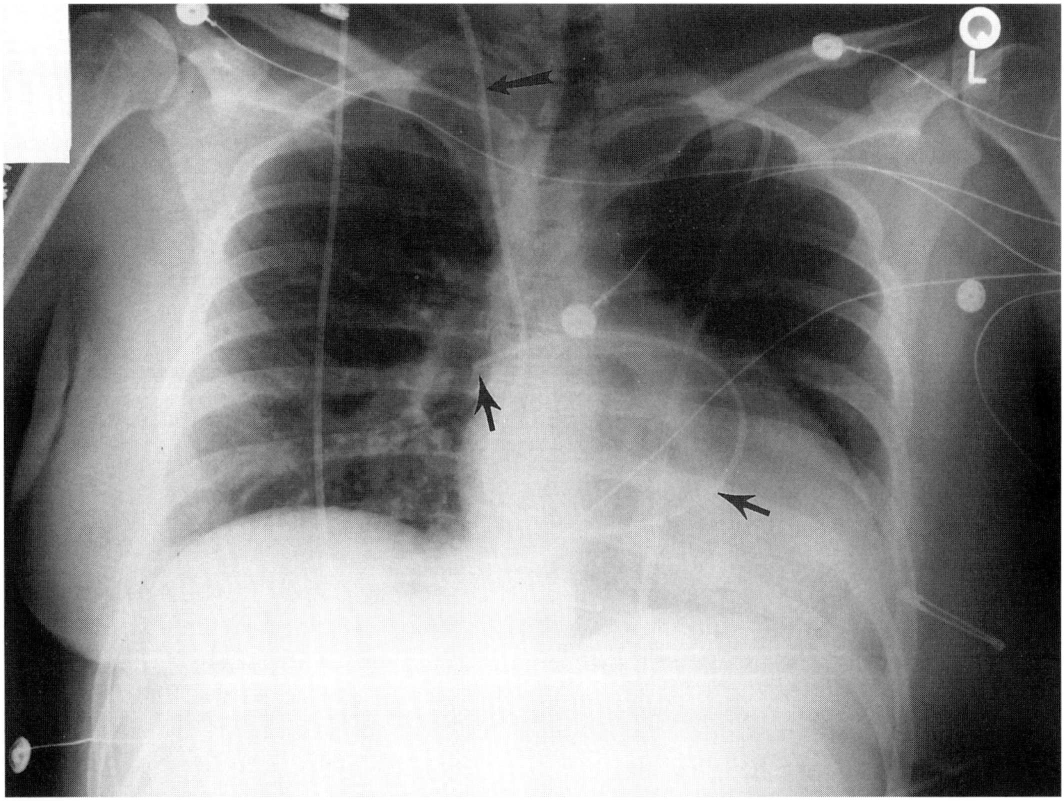

Fig. 3-31 The pulmonary artery catheter enters the right atrium, passes through the tricuspid valve into the right ventricle, and exits the pulmonic valve into the main pulmonary artery. An arrow marks the tip of the catheter. Notice that the catheter does not extend past the medial third of the hemithorax. This patient has primary pulmonary hypertension (notice the increased size of the pulmonary arteries) and a permanent Hickman catheter in place for continuous infusion of a pulmonary artery vasodilator.

position changes. Heart sounds are consistent with congestive heart failure; S_4 or S_3 gallop rhythm and murmurs are often present. Hemodynamic changes include decreased cardiac output, increased pulmonary capillary wedge pressure, and with biventricular failure, increased right heart pressures. Tachycardia and hypotension are common. Most patients have some degree of hypoxemia.

Radiologic Appearance

In early cardiogenic pulmonary edema the nurse observes an opaque "butterfly" pattern on the chest radiograph that results from pulmonary artery congestion in the hilar area. The heart is enlarged, and the pulmonary arteries and veins are prominent. The chest radiograph demonstrates a diffuse interstitial pattern (engorgement of perivascular and peribronchial interstitial tissues from fluid backup) followed by an alveolar pattern that ascends from the bases and does not usually involve the apices. The degree of fluid overload determines the height of the interstitial and alveolar patterns. Kerley lines are present if the intralobular septa are thickened. Sometimes the nurse observes *cephalization*, an increase in the size and visibility of pulmonary vessels near the apices. As the alveoli fill with fluid, atelectasis also may occur (Fig. 3-32).

Nursing Implications

Patients with cardiogenic pulmonary edema need normovolemia, which is usually achieved with fluid restriction and medications such as morphine, diuretics, vasodilators, inotropes, afterload or preload agents, or contractility agents. These patients also require supplemental oxygen and elevation of the head of the bed. Patients with severe cardiogenic pulmonary edema may require intraaortic balloon pumping for diastolic augmentation of the left ventricle.

NONCARDIOGENIC PULMONARY EDEMA: (ADULT RESPIRATORY DISTRESS SYNDROME)

Definition

Adult respiratory distress syndrome (ARDS) is pulmonary edema with normal cardiac function; it is not the result of increased hydrostatic pressure but

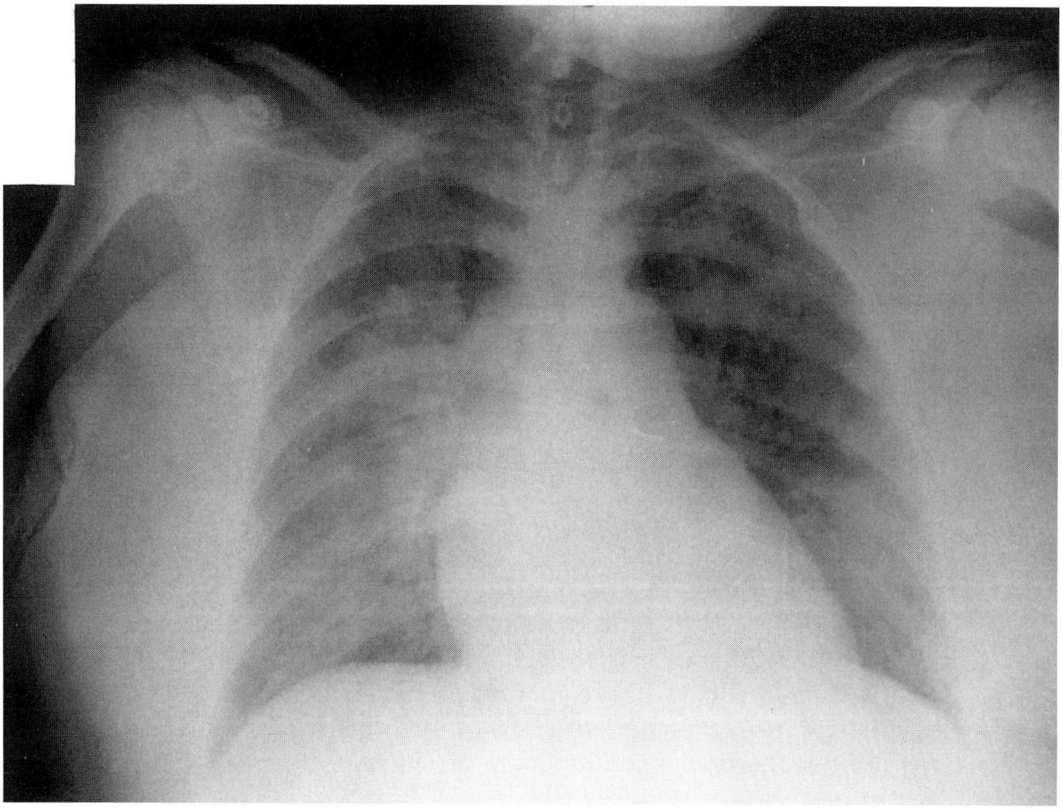

Fig. 3-32 Cardiogenic pulmonary edema is present in this patient. An enlarged heart and a relative sparing of infiltrates from the upper lung fields can be seen.

of altered permeability coefficient (Starling's law). The alveolar capillary membrane is injured from either the airway (local) or the blood (systemic) side. Local lung injury (such as aspiration, near drowning, pneumonia, smoke inhalation, or pulmonary contusion) or systemic lung injury (such as fractures, sepsis, shock, or multiple blood transfusions) may precipitate ARDS.

Clinical Findings

Early in ARDS the patient complains of dyspnea and increased work of breathing, which often requires intubation and mechanical ventilation. There is tachypnea with normal-to-small tidal volumes, grunting, diaphoresis, intercostal retractions, and sometimes cyanosis. Lungs that are initially clear develop crackles throughout. The crackles do not move with changes in patient position as in cardiogenic pulmonary edema. The pulmonary capillary wedge pressure is normal to low. Arterial blood gases demonstrate hypoxemia that is often refractory to supplemental oxygen (shunt).

Radiologic Appearance

Regardless of patient position there are bilateral, diffuse, fluffy infiltrates on the chest radiograph. The infiltrates generally affect both the bases and the apices of the left and right lungs equally and are not dependent on position. Often all five lobes are affected. The heart and pulmonary vessels are normal size (Fig. 3-33).

Nursing Implications

There is no direct treatment for ARDS; all interventions are supportive. In general, attempts are made to keep the patient normovolemic; fluid overload encourages fluid to leave the capillary and enter the alveoli, which are already overcome with fluid and debris. This is often difficult in the acute trauma patient who requires volume repletion and in all patients requiring parenteral antibiotics, vasoactive drips, and nutrition. Administration of supplemental oxygen and positive-end expiratory pressure aids in oxygenating tissues without inducing oxygen toxicity. Therapies currently under investigation include extracorporeal or intravenous oxygenators and surfactant repletion.

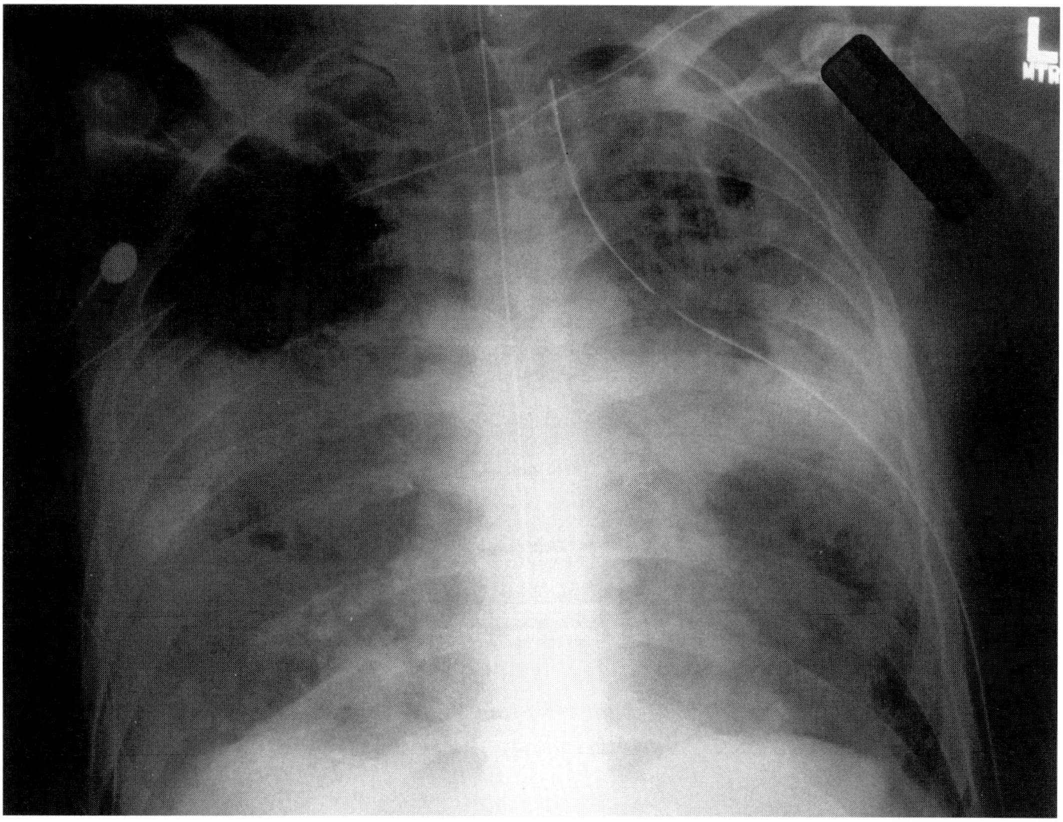

Fig. 3-33 This is an example of adult respiratory distress syndrome (ARDS), noncardiogenic pulmonary edema. Notice the diffuse bilateral infiltrates and a normal-sized heart.

PULMONARY EMBOLISM

Definition

Pulmonary embolism is an obstruction to blood flow in a pulmonary artery or capillary. The obstruction is a thrombus that usually develops in the deep veins of the legs or pelvis or from the right side of the heart, breaking loose to travel to the lungs. Other types of pulmonary emboli include air, amniotic fluid, fat, foreign bodies, parasitic or septic emboli, or tumor fragments. Stasis of blood flow, injury to the intima of the blood vessel, and alterations in the coagulation-fibrinolytic system predispose the blood to form a thrombus. Risk factors for development of pulmonary embolism include atrial fibrillation, birth control pills, burns, cancer of the chest or abdomen, chronic pulmonary disease, immobility, trauma, obesity, pregnancy, varicose veins, and surgery. A pulmonary embolism reduces the size of the pulmonary vascular bed and increases pulmonary vascular resistance and pulmonary artery pressure. Sometimes the right ventricular workload is increased, possibly causing failure.

Clinical Findings

Typical findings of deep-vein thrombosis include tenderness, redness, warmth, and edema of the involved extremity. Development of a pulmonary embolism also causes various degrees of one or more of the following symptoms: tachypnea, pleuritic chest pain, acute anxiety, diaphoresis, cough, nausea, hypoxemia, tachycardia, and hemoptysis. The nurse may also assess a few wheezes or crackles, dullness to percussion when a concomitant pleural effusion is present, or a pleural friction rub with infarction. Impedance plethysmography, echocardiography, or ultrasonography may be positive for deep-vein or heart chamber clot formation. An electrocardiogram may show strain on the right side of the heart or pulmonary hypertension in large or multiple pulmonary emboli. Arterial blood gases are not specific and may show respiratory alkalosis from tachypnea and anxiety or hypoxemia.

Radiologic Appearance

A pulmonary embolism is often not recognizable on a chest radiograph, making the diagnosis slightly more difficult. As surfactant is destroyed, small areas of atelectasis or an infiltrate develop. If a pulmonary embolus is present in a large pulmonary artery, the nurse may see the pulmonary artery truncate or stop at the level of the embolus. If a pulmonary infarct has occurred, there may be "tenting," or a wedge-shaped infiltrate, often near the diaphragm and a pleural effusion. Septic emboli appear as multiple, small, round or irregularly-shaped shaggy densities.

When a pulmonary embolism is suspected, the physician will usually order a ventilation-perfusion scan to be performed. This test compares the amount of perfusion in a lung segment to the amount of ventilation in that segment. In healthy people, ventilation and perfusion are matched. With a pulmonary embolism, ventilation is normal but perfusion is decreased or absent in the affected lung segments. Segmental or larger perfusion defects with normal ventilation and a normal chest radiograph indicate a high probability that pulmonary embolism has occurred.

In the critically ill patient, especially in one receiving mechanical ventilation therapy, ventilation-perfusion scans are often suboptimal. The ventilation component of the test cannot be easily performed on patients receiving continuous mechanical ventilation. Ventilation-perfusion scans are more difficult to interpret in patients with lung diseases such as pneumonia because of altered ventilation or perfusion. Unfortunately, many ventilation-perfusion scans are not absolutely diagnostic and result in the performance of pulmonary angiography.

A pulmonary angiogram is the "gold standard" for diagnosing pulmonary embolism. It is performed in all patients who have a high index of suspicion for pulmonary embolism and who have an indeterminate or low-probability ventilation-perfusion scan. Unfortunately, the angiogram is associated with many risks, which makes physicians reluctant to order it. The risks of the test are weighed against confirmation of the diagnosis of pulmonary embolism and prolonged systemic anticoagulation. Patients with renal insufficiency may not be eligible for angiography or venography because of the radiopaque dye required for the test. A positive angiogram shows filling defects (narrow lumen) of the blood vessel or an abrupt vessel cutoff (truncation).

A vena caval filter is inserted in patients who are unable to undergo long-term anticoagulation and who have a positive test for deep-vein thrombosis or pulmonary embolism. A vena caval filter looks like a small wire umbrella or parachute and is inserted into the inferior vena cava through the femoral vein. Physicians who strongly suspect pulmonary embolism but who are unable to diagnose it may elect to insert a filter into the inferior vena cava to protect the patient from future pulmonary embolism (Figs. 3-34, 3-35, 3-36, 3-37, and 3-38).

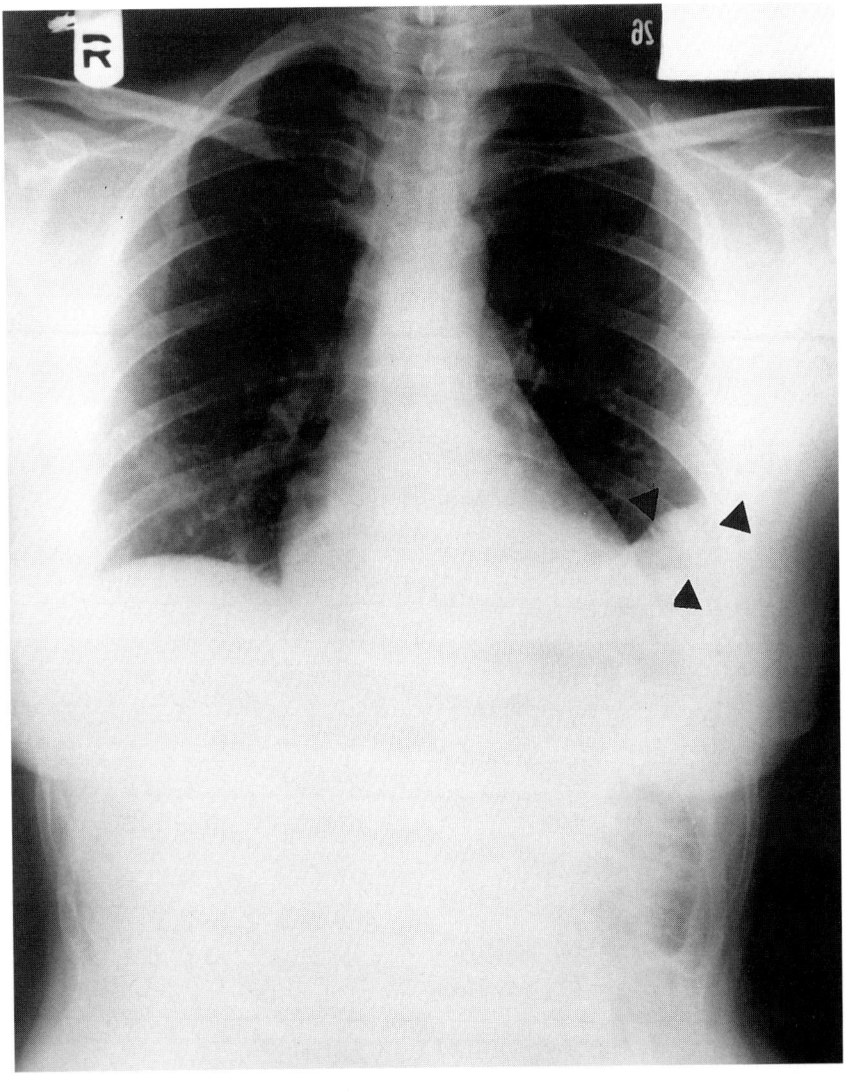

Fig. 3-34 This radiograph has a fairly classic sign of pulmonary infarction. Notice the tenting on the left diaphragm at the outer edge of the heart. Some physicians term this sign a "buffalo hump."

A

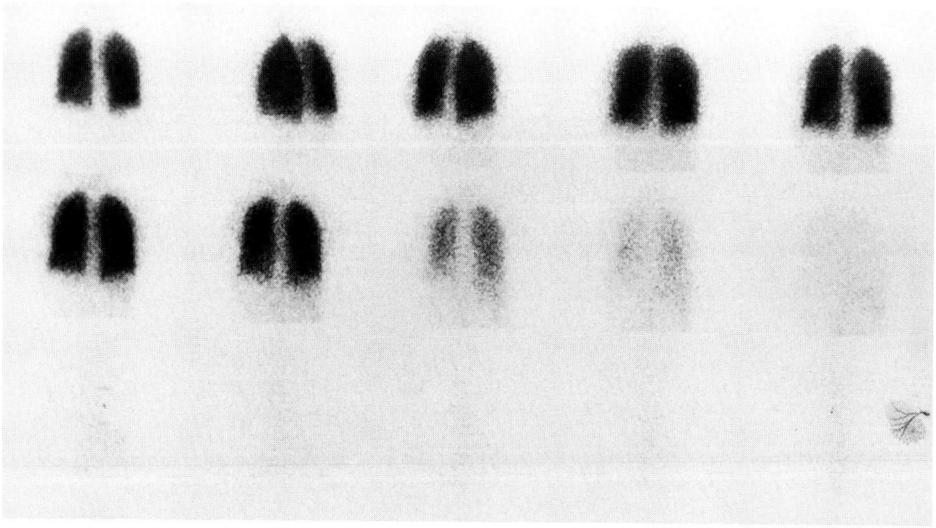

B

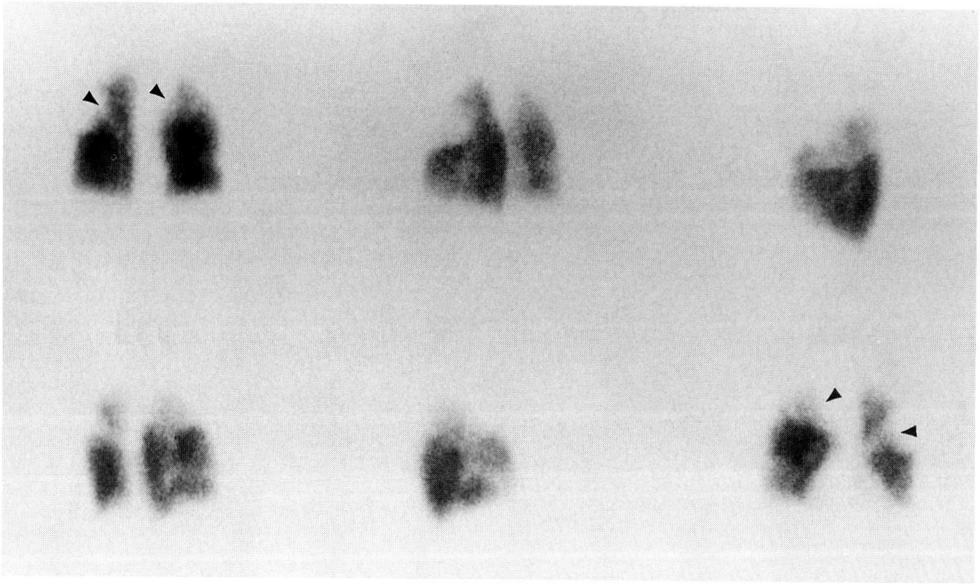

Fig. 3-35 Ventilation-perfusion scan. **A,** Ventilation. **B,** Perfusion. Although ventilation is essentially normal, perfusion to many areas of the lung is absent. The multiple mismatched segments indicate a high probability of pulmonary embolism.

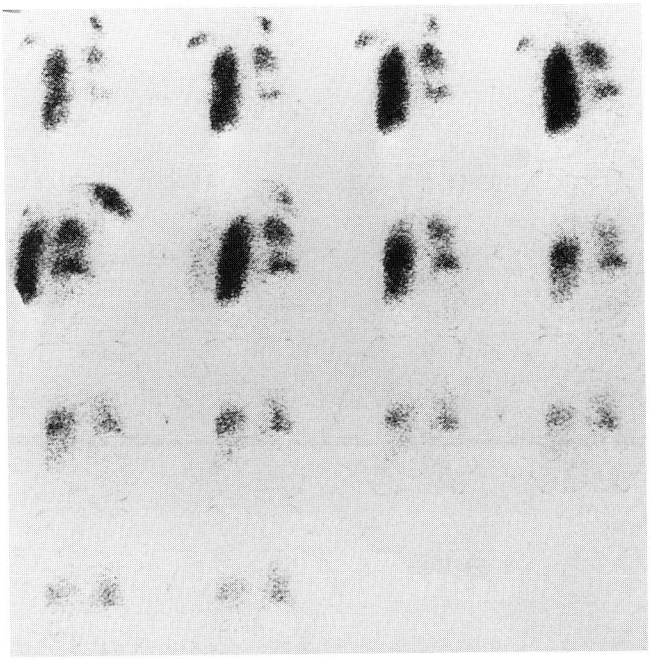

A

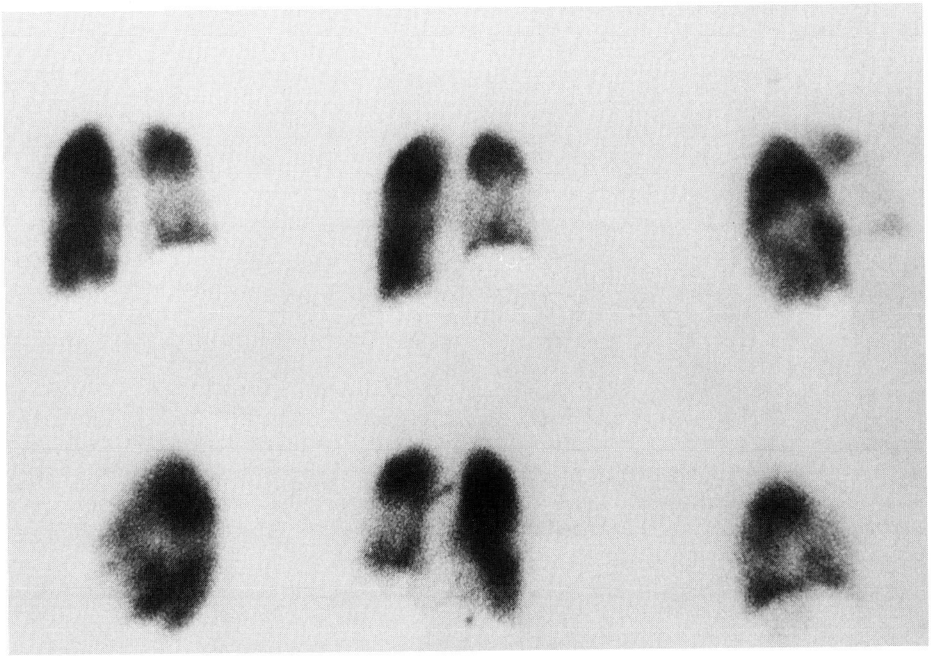

B

Fig. 3-36 This is an example of an indeterminate or negative ventilation-perfusion (V/Q) scan. There are not mismatched segments of ventilation and perfusion.

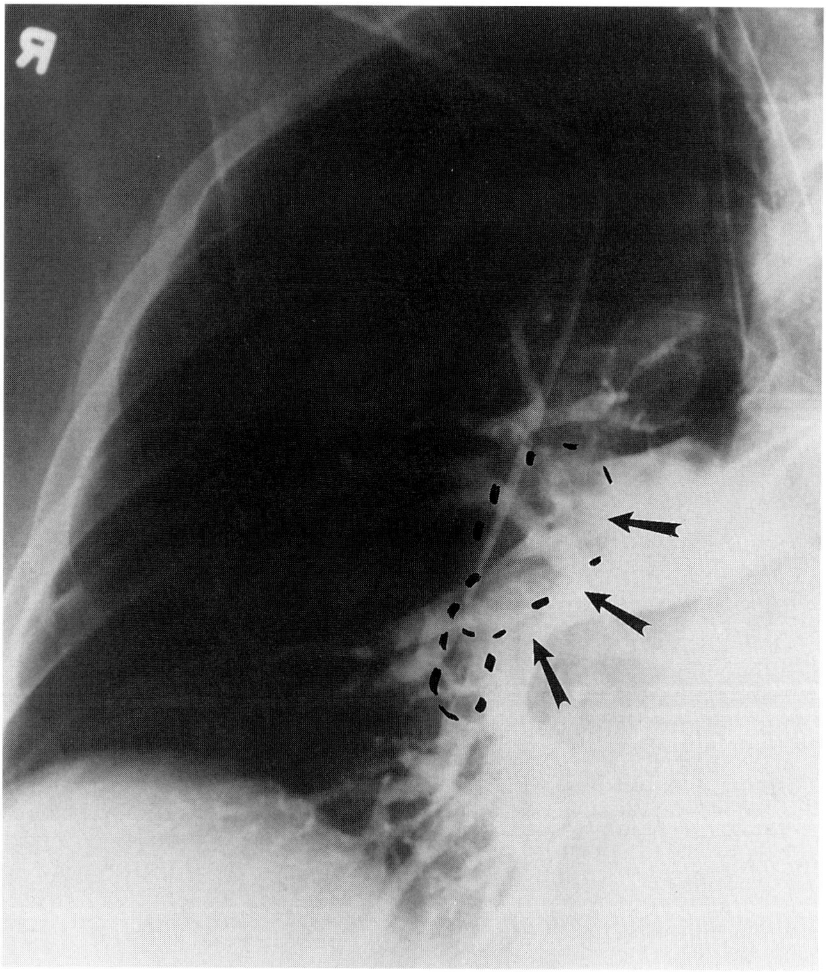

Fig. 3-37 An angiogram is suggestive of a pulmonary embolism when there is scalloping or narrowing of a branch of the pulmonary artery. The defect is highlighted by arrows and outlined with dashes.

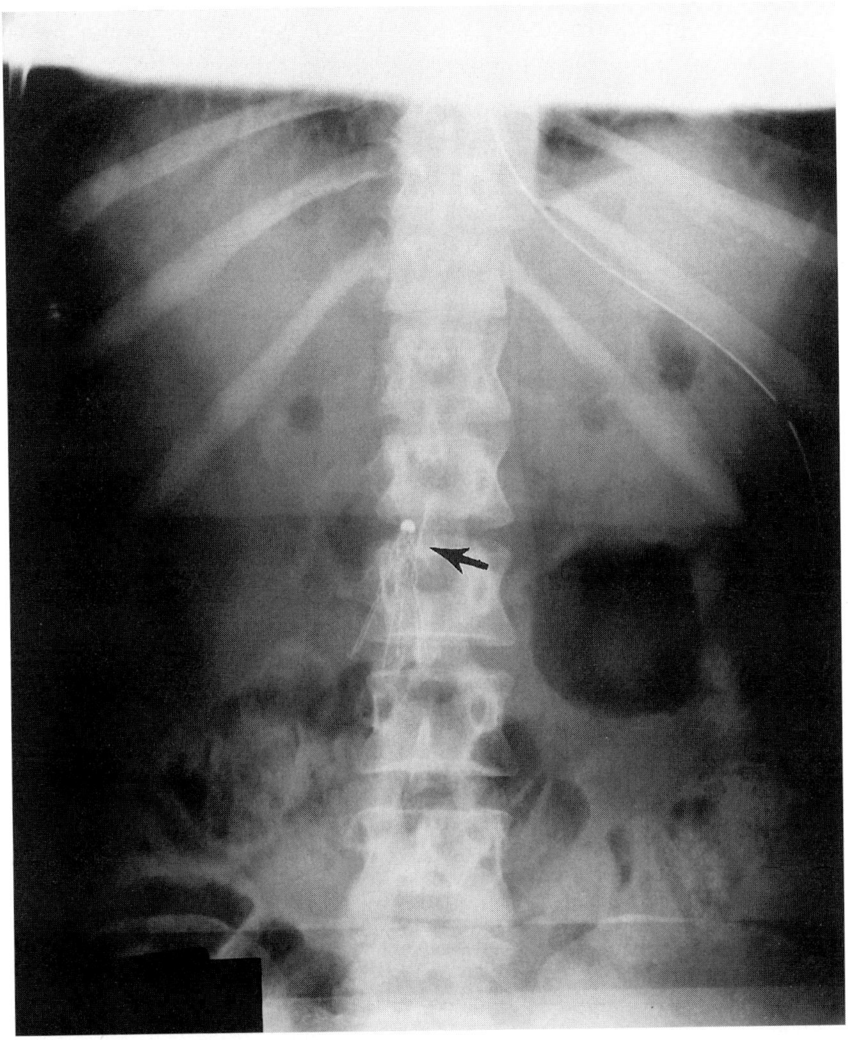

Fig. 3-38 This radiograph shows an umbrella filter in the patient's inferior vena cava. Notice the wires with hooks under the diaphragm in the inferior vena cava. This patient also has a nasogastric tube in place.

Nursing Implications

Patients who are at high risk for deep-vein thrombosis (DVT) or pulmonary embolism should be observed closely. In many instances the problem can be prevented by administering a low dose of heparin or warfarin, using proper positioning, encouraging activity, applying and using pneumatic compression devices, immobilizing fractures, and removing/inserting intravenous catheters properly. When it does occur, the treatment is supportive in most cases. The nurse should first focus on reestablishing normal oxygenation and relieving chest pain when it occurs. Interventions may include nasal oxygen or mechanical ventilation. If the pulmonary embolism is life threatening, the physician may order administration of thrombolytic agents to the patient.

LUNG RESECTION AND PNEUMONECTOMY

Definition

Lung resection is the removal of a segment or lobe of the lung. A pneumonectomy is the removal of an entire lung. Tumors, persistent air leaks, and bullae are common reasons for performing a lung resection.

Clinical Findings

Nursing assessments vary with the amount of lung resected. Any time a scar is found on the thorax, the nurse should ask the patient what type of surgical procedure was performed. In many instances the nurse will not be able to appreciate differences in lung volumes with traditional chest assessment techniques. The nurse may observe asymmetrical lung expansion or dullness to percussion with lobar or multilobar resection. Tachypnea may be observed. With a pneumonectomy there is no air movement on the affected side, although the other lung may expand and “herniate” into the affected side, causing some air movement. There is dullness to percussion over the affected side, and no breath sounds are usually heard unless the opposite lung has sufficiently enlarged.

Radiologic Appearance

The radiologic picture is varied. Depending on what segment or lobe is removed, the nurse may be able to identify a change on the chest radiograph.

Wire clips or sutures where the bronchus and larger pulmonary arteries have been tied off are often visible. The nurse may identify what appears to be collapse, but is actually postoperative consolidation of tissue. When the patient has had a pneumonectomy there is usually no air on the surgical side, but there are clips that tie off the mainstem bronchus and pulmonary arteries. Sometimes following pneumonectomy the other lung will expand beyond its usual boundaries and cross over the midline (Fig. 3-39).

Nursing Implications

The nurse should remember that removal of a segment or lobe often changes the anatomical position of the airways, thus chest physical therapy positions often need to be altered to aid in the drainage of a lung abscess or infiltrate. Sometimes the nurse will be able to identify these changes on the chest radiograph, especially if both a PA and a lateral projection are available.

LUNG TRANSPLANTATION

Definition

Lung transplantation is the removal of a patient's lung and insertion of a donor lung. Only about 200 lung transplants are performed annually because of a shortage of donors. The pathologic conditions that lead to lung transplantation include severe restrictive conditions (such as interstitial pulmonary fibrosis), obstructive (such as emphysema, bronchitis, cystic fibrosis), or vascular (such as primary pulmonary hypertension) lung disease. In most cases only one lung is replaced; however, transplant may involve a heart and one lung, both lungs, or both lungs and a heart depending on the pathologic conditions. Two main problems in lung transplantation are rejection and infection. Often the two occur simultaneously, and both increase the risk of morbidity and mortality.

Clinical Findings

Lung transplant patients are challenging and offer diverse clinical findings. The noninfected, nonrejecting lung transplant patient has the clinical findings of a healthy patient with a few exceptions. Immunosuppression causes a Cushingoid appearance (moon face, buffalo hump on the back of the neck, truncal obesity, muscular atrophy, etc.). The nurse assesses findings consis-

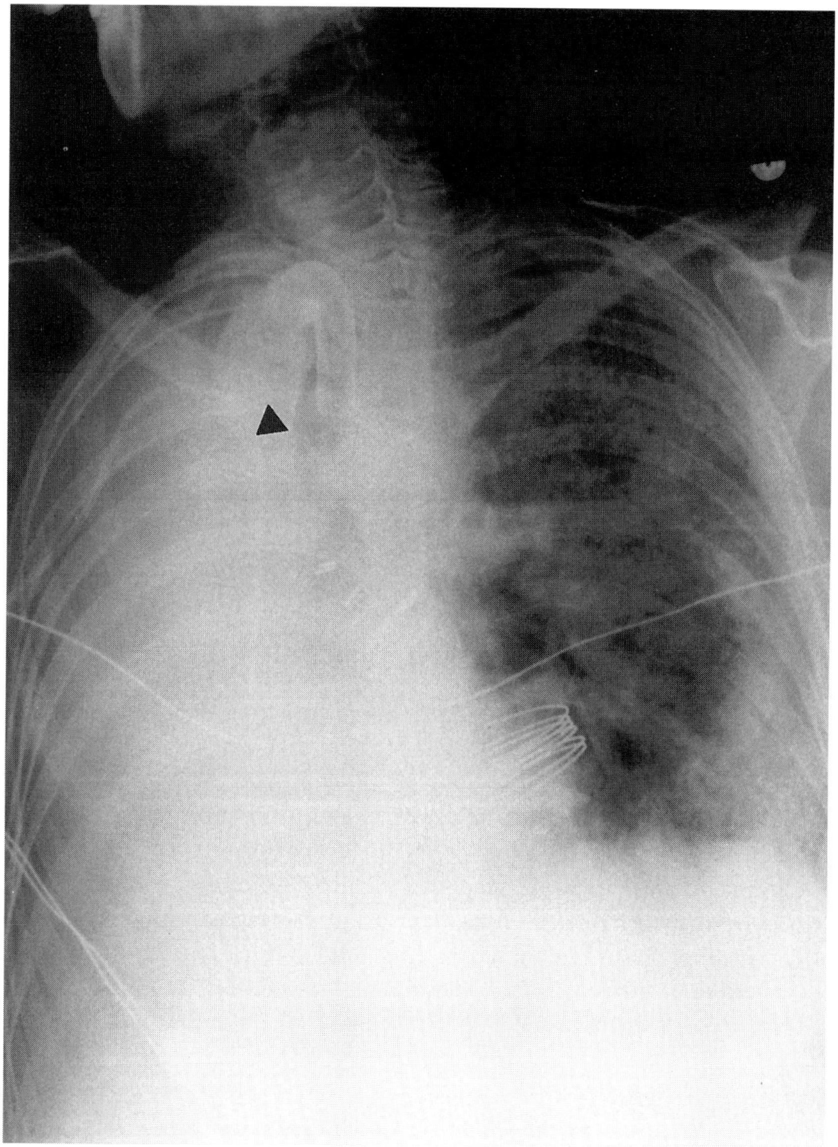

Fig. 3-39 A pneumonectomy is the absence of one lung. Bronchial clips can be viewed in this radiograph. Many times the remaining lung will enlarge in size to accommodate patient requirements.

tent with the disease process in the native lung. When infection or rejection occurs, the patient may have a 0.5°F (.2 to .3°C) increase in temperature, a 1% to 2% decrease in arterial saturation through pulse oximetry, or increased dyspnea. The patient may also complain of cough or sputum production.

Radiologic Appearance

The chest radiograph of a patient with a transplanted lung is interesting to see. With single lung or single lung and heart transplantation, the native lung has the characteristics of the disease process leading to transplantation. The native lung commonly has changes consistent with interstitial fibrosis or emphysema. With interstitial fibrosis there is an interstitial pattern with Kerley lines or honeycombing, and the lung appears small in size. With emphysema the native lung is hyperinflated from air-trapping with a flattened diaphragm and few vascular markings. The transplanted lung appears normal, but the nurse may see vascular clips or sutures in the hilar region at the pulmonary artery anastomosis and wire clips or sutures at the level of the bronchial anastomosis. If the patient develops infection in the transplanted lung, there is usually an infiltrate present. With rejection the patient develops an alveolar or interstitial pattern on the chest radiograph (Fig. 3-40).

Nursing Implications

If infection or rejection occur, the lung transplant patient requires prompt, accurate care to preserve the transplanted lung. The nurse should be prepared to administer therapeutic doses of immunosuppressive agents or antirejection agents to treat rejection and antibiotics, antifungal agents, or antiviral agents to treat infection. The nurse must remember that opportunistic microorganisms such as cytomegalovirus (CMV) and pneumocystis are common causes of infection. Infected patients often require supplemental oxygen through a nasal cannula and chest physical therapy.

LUNG TUMORS

Definition

Lung tumors may appear anywhere in the lung and may involve the lymphatic system. In general, adenocarcinomas and large-cell carcinomas are seen in the peripheral lung and squamous-cell carcinomas are found in the

A

B

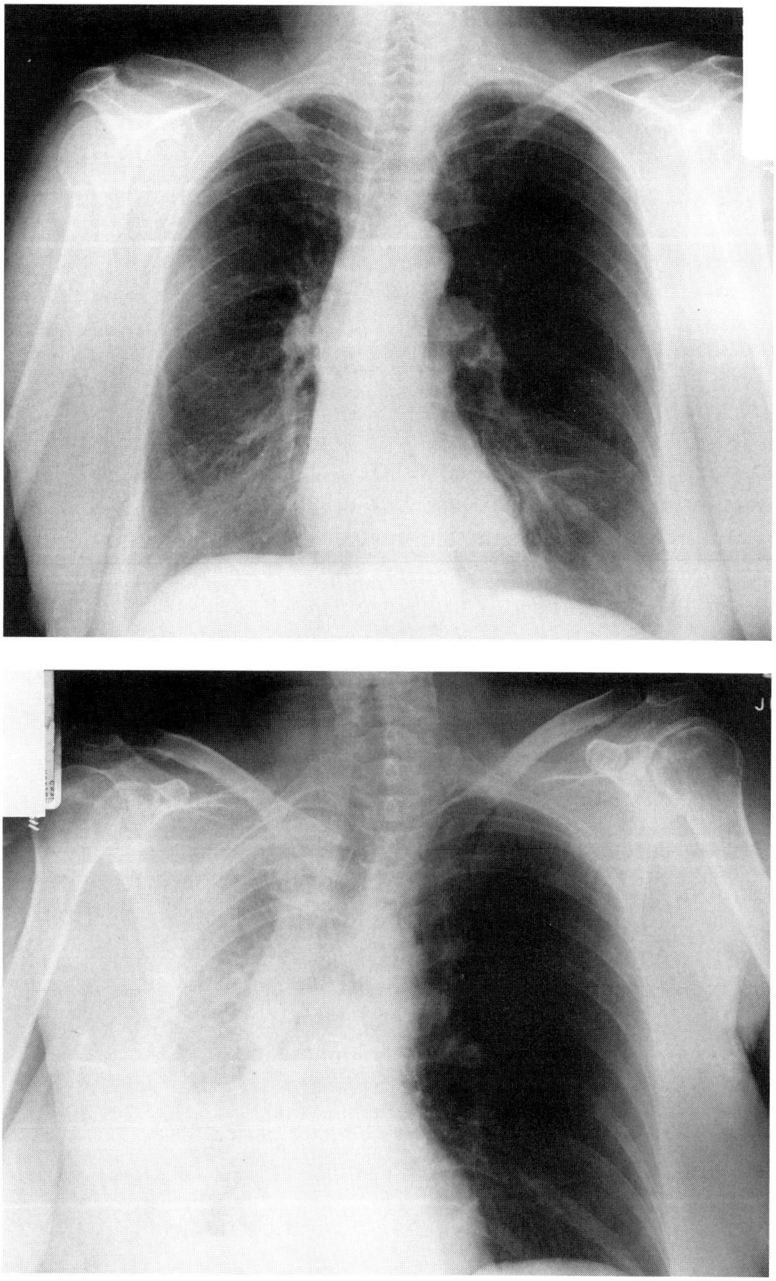

Fig. 3-40 These two films are of a patient following lung transplantation. Notice the clips in the right mid-central lung field. **A,** Normal postopcrative film. The right lung is the transplanted lung, and the left lung has severe emphysema. **B,** Right lung rejection. Notice the diffuse infiltrates and small lung volume compared to the previous radiograph.

central regions. Rapidly growing small-cell carcinomas develop proximally and metastasize early. Squamous-cell carcinomas account for the majority of tumors and other metastases to the hilar area.

Clinical Findings

Most patients complain of dyspnea, cough, hemoptysis, chest pain, or weight loss. The patient may also have nausea, vomiting, weakness, dysphagia, superior vena caval syndrome, hoarseness, or headache. The patient may have been admitted with physical signs and symptoms of pneumonia that were precipitated by an inability to clear secretions past the tumor. In most cases the chest examination is unremarkable; there may be evidence of a pleural effusion or localized wheezing from airway obstruction.

Radiologic Appearance

A tumor appears as an opaque density, often round and ranging in size from a few millimeters to 4 to 5 cm. If the tumor is a large-cell carcinoma, there may be a cavity, often located in the upper lung fields. A cavity appears as a thin, white ring with a hyperlucent center. In some instances there may be fullness in the hilar region, or enlarged lymph nodes may be seen alongside the trachea as opaque "bumps." It is important for the nurse to try to determine the position of the tumor in relation to large airways and vascular structures (Figs. 3-41 and 3-42).

Nursing Implications

Patients undergoing tumor evaluation will require multiple procedures, including thoracentesis, bronchoscopy, and CT scans. Once the diagnosis is made, the patient may require surgery or administration of chemotherapy agents. The patient needs much education and support throughout this process.

HEART VALVES

Definition

Patients with severe tricuspid, pulmonic, mitral, or aortic valve insufficiency or stenosis require removal of the diseased valve and insertion of a prosthetic

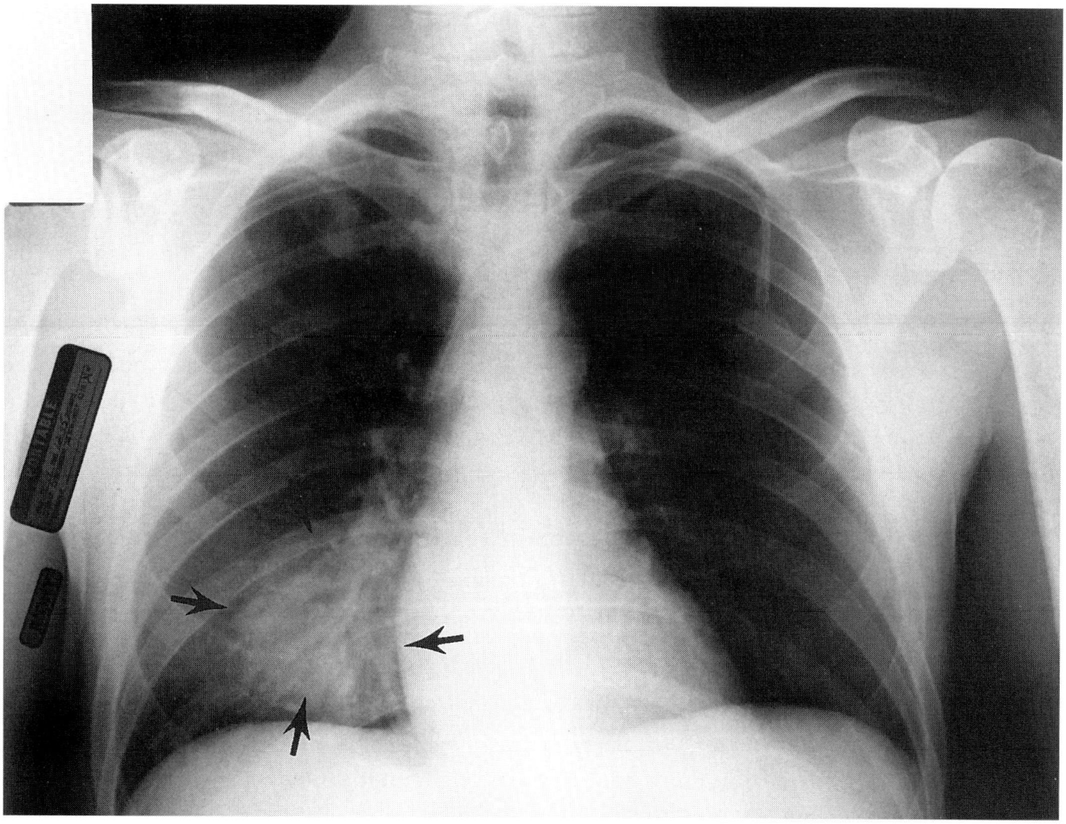

Fig. 3-41 This radiograph demonstrates a large inoperable central tumor resulting from chronic obstructive lung disease.

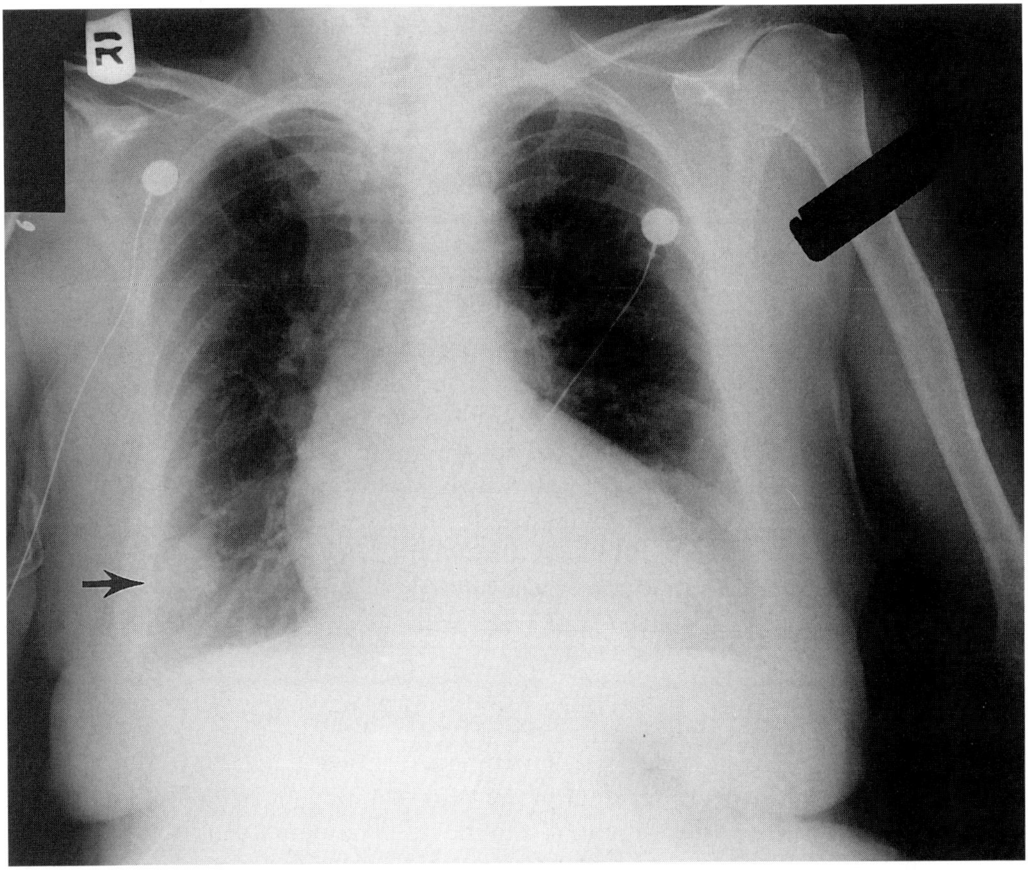

Fig. 3-42 This patient has a large inoperable peripheral tumor resulting from chronic obstructive lung disease.

valve. The type of valve inserted depends on physician preferences and regional differences in patient care. The most common valves are the St. Jude and the Medtronic. Also available is the Starr Edwards, porcine Hancok, and foreign-used Bjork Shiley. Each of these valves has a different appearance on the chest radiograph.

Clinical Findings

Patients requiring replacement of heart valves generally have signs of chronic cardiac failure. The patient often experiences low cardiac output, abnormal heart tones, dyspnea, and dysrhythmias. After valve replacement the patient often has normal assessment findings.

Radiologic Appearance

On a chest radiograph, a valve is almost always recognized by a metallic ring. The exception is the porcine valve, which may not be visible on a chest radiograph. The Medtronic valve has a visible Y-shaped center that represents the valve leaflets; two projections may be seen in the center of the St. Jude valve, especially on a lateral chest radiograph; and the Starr Edwards valve has a ring with a cup and a plastic ball, which is often not visible. The aortic valve is seen at the root of the aorta on the left side of the chest. Located just below the aortic valve is the mitral valve, also on the left side of the chest. These two valves may appear to intersect. On the right side of the chest are the pulmonic (superior) and the tricuspid (inferior) valves (Figs. 3-43, 3-44, and 3-45).

Nursing Implications

As with all invasive devices, the nurse should notify the physician if a valve suddenly appears to be out of place. Often the patient will develop symptoms that suggest malfunctioning of the valves. The nurse should also teach the patient about dental prophylaxis and anticoagulation.

VENTRICULAR ASSIST DEVICE

Definition

A ventricular assist device (VAD) is primarily used after cardiothoracic surgery to assume the work of pumping blood from one or both ineffectively

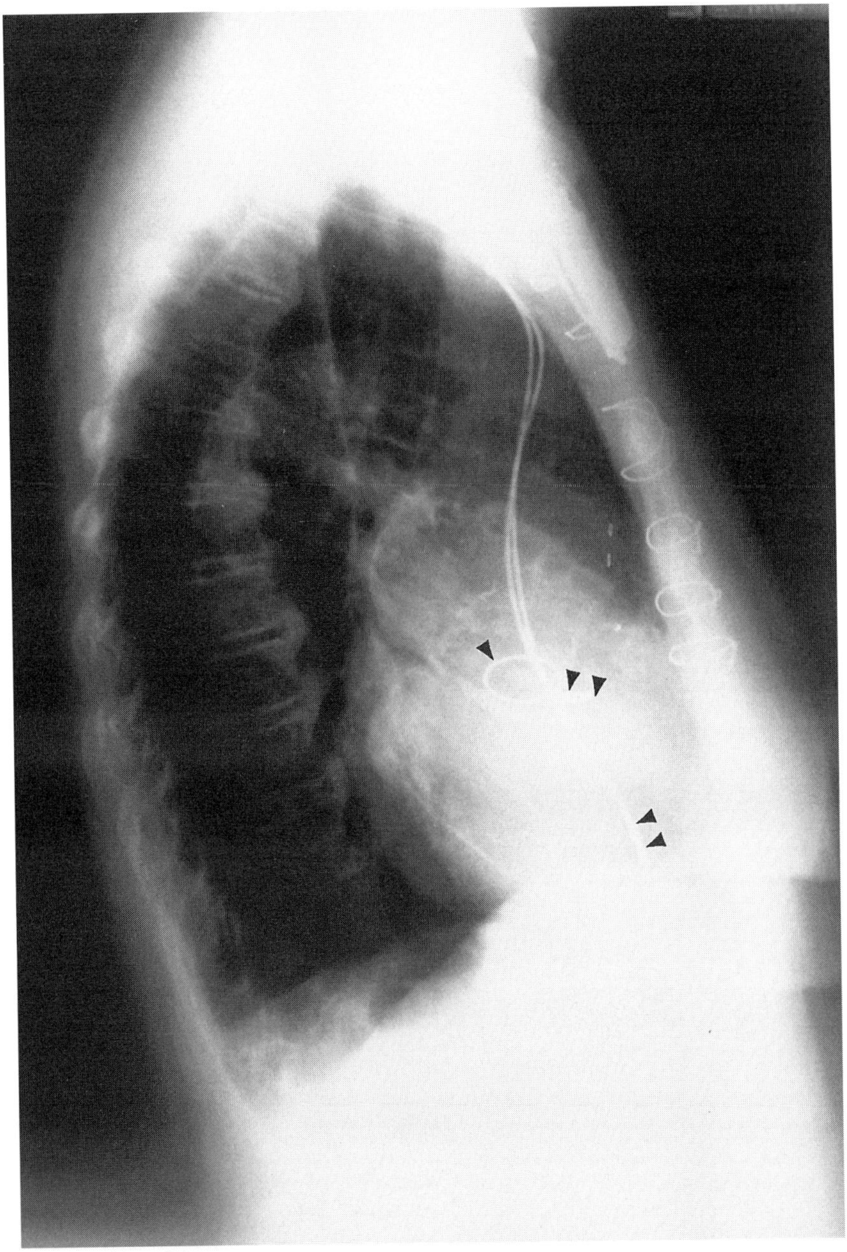

Fig. 3-43 This radiograph illustrates the normal position of an artificial aortic valve.

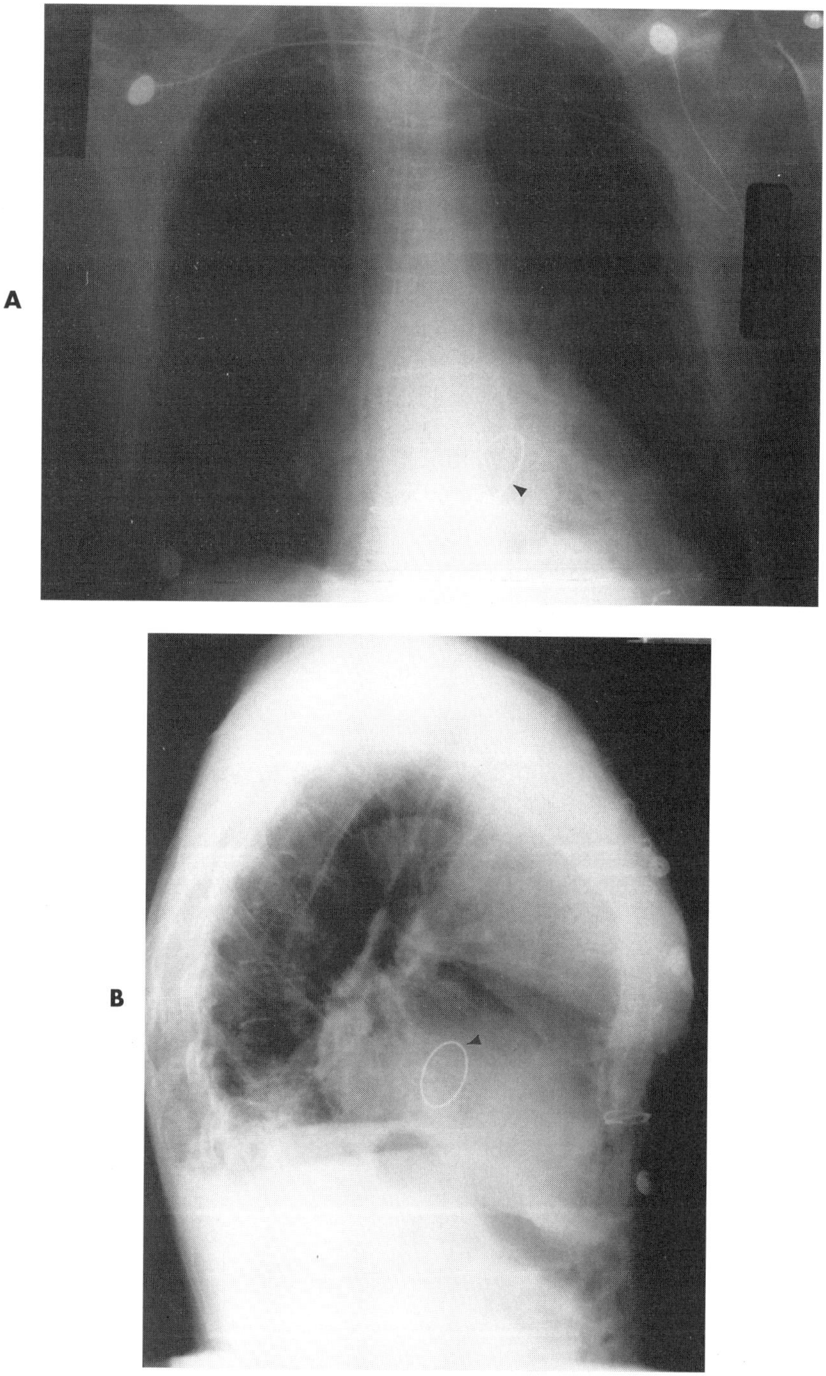

Fig. 3-44 **A** and **B,** These radiographs illustrate the normal position of an artificial mitral valve.

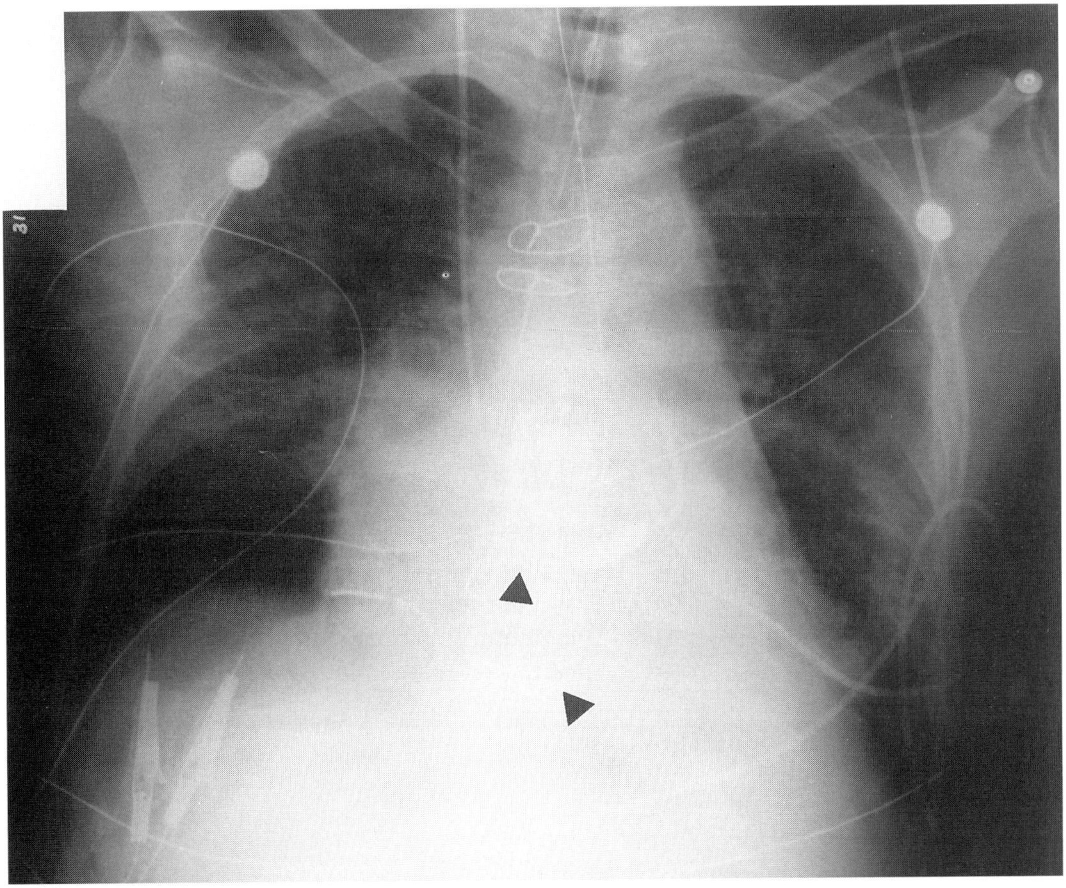

Fig. 3-45 Tricuspid valve replacements are rarely performed. This radiograph illustrates the normal position of an artificial tricuspid valve. Notice the correct position of an endotracheal tube, two mediastinal chest tubes, a right internal jugular catheter, a nasogastric tube, and pacer wires with alligator clips.

contracting ventricles. A large-bore catheter or tube is inserted surgically into either the left or right ventricle and connected to a machine that performs the work of the ventricle. The term *RVAD* or *LVAD* is used when the device is inserted into the right or left ventricle, respectively. Some patients require simultaneous insertion of biventricular assist devices (BIVAD).

Clinical Findings

Patients requiring VAD insertion have severe cardiac dysfunction. They are generally hypotensive with low cardiac output. The patient is usually sent to surgery with low cardiac output, shock, cyanosis, and diminished heart tones following acute myocardial infarction. In some cases the VAD is placed in the operating room during cardiothoracic surgery when the team is unable to wean the patient from the bypass machine.

Radiologic Appearance

Two large plastic hoses can be seen entering or emerging from an enlarged heart on the chest radiograph (Fig. 3-46).

Nursing Implications

Patients with a VAD require anticoagulation and sedation. In many cases the VAD is a bridge to cardiac transplant.

WIDENED MEDIASTINUM

Definition

There are several causes of a widened mediastinum. The most common causes seen in an intensive care unit or emergency department are aortic aneurysm or rupture and large tumor or lymph nodes.

There is a high mortality rate associated with aortic rupture. Most patients die before arriving in the emergency department; a small percentage, less than 10%, are discharged from the hospital. A widened mediastinum and aortic injury are often associated with first or second rib fracture, high sternal fracture, or left clavicular fracture. Complete or partial dissection of the aorta usually results from a deceleration injury such as a motor vehicle accident. Tears in the aorta occur at points of anatomic fixation; the most common site

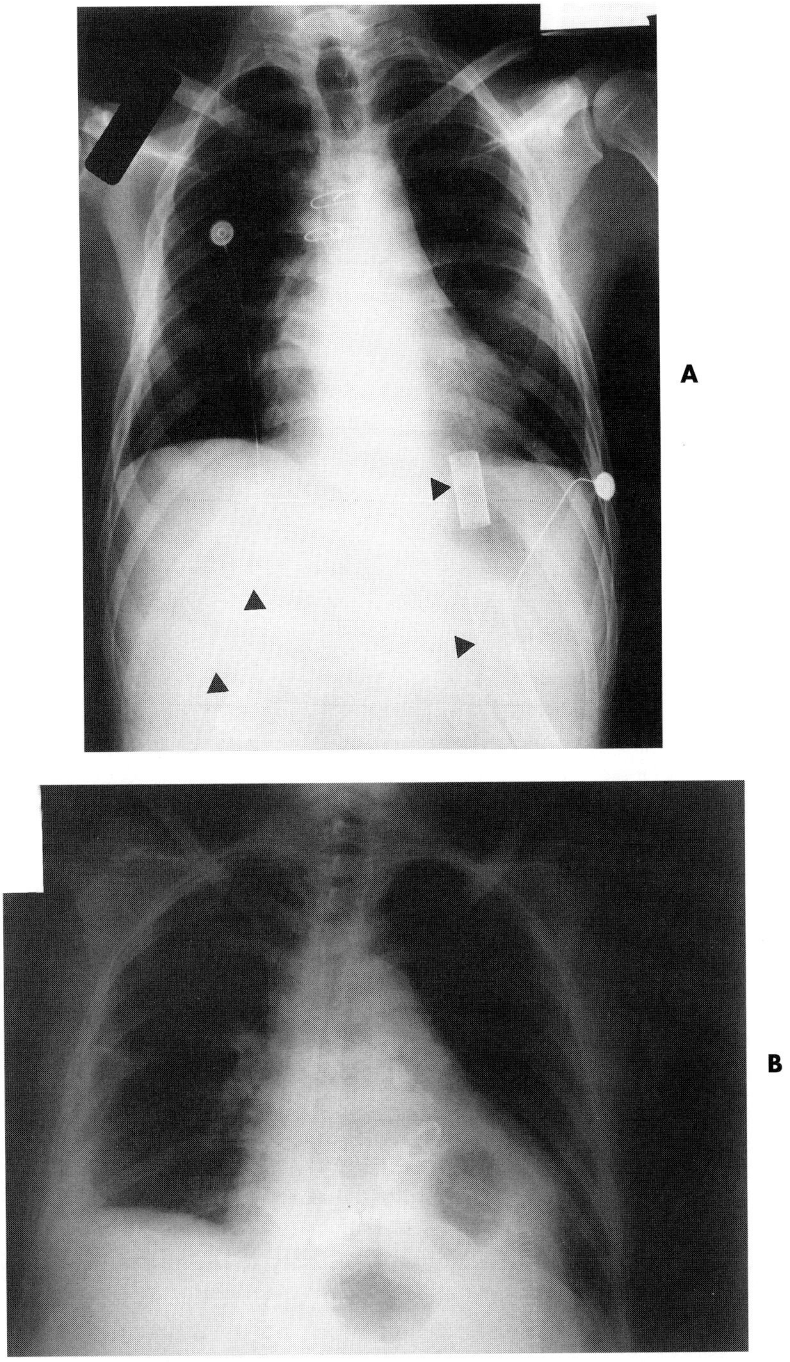

Fig. 3-46 Ventricular assist devices (VADs) have several appearances. **A,** One example of a VAD with large tubes extending from the heart and abdomen. **B,** Notice the presence of the valves and atelectasis.

is distal to the left subclavian artery on the descending thoracic aorta. Tears may also occur on the ascending aorta at the pericardial sac and at the diaphragm as the aorta enters the abdomen. On deceleration the intima and media of the vessel tear and the adventitia balloons into a pseudoaneurysm.

Large mediastinal tumors or lymph nodes are usually malignant and inoperable; some respond well to radiation therapy and chemotherapy, but the mortality rate is usually high. The patient may develop superior vena caval syndrome, which impedes drainage from head, upper thorax, and upper extremities. This results in decreased venous return and increased venous pressure.

Clinical Findings

Aortic aneurysm is associated with patient complaints of sternal or interscapular back pain, dyspnea, or hoarseness that is the result of hematoma pressure around the aortic arch. Some patients have upper extremity hypertension but most have general hypotension (shock) secondary to hypovolemia. The femoral or radial pulse is absent or delayed, and there is a precordial or interscapular murmur as a result of turbulence across the disrupted area. Most patients have some degree of lower-extremity neuromuscular or sensory deficit. The nurse may observe tachypnea or cyanosis, and the patient may develop cardiopulmonary arrest at any time. A blood count will show low hemoglobin and hematocrit and arterial blood gases will generally demonstrate hypoxemia with respiratory alkalosis or acidosis.

Patients with superior vena caval syndrome complain of dyspnea, chest pain, headache, and cough. There may also be complaints of recent vision changes and lethargy. Patients with superior vena caval syndrome have generalized upper-body edema involving the arms, neck, thorax above the nipple line, and head. Thoracic and neck veins are distended. The lower extremities are of normal size.

Radiologic Appearance

With a ruptured aorta or aortic aneurysm the radiograph shows a widened mediastinum on a film taken with the patient in an upright or supine position. A massive pleural effusion is present with a ruptured aorta and is more commonly observed in the left hemithorax; the entire left side of the chest may be opacified. The trachea and esophagus are often deviated (pushed) to the right side by the pleural effusion. An aortogram confirms aortic injury and a CT scan is useful in superior vena caval syndrome to locate tumor or lymph nodes (Figs. 3-47 and 3-48).

Nursing Implications

The nurse should always be ready to perform cardiopulmonary resuscitation, especially during angiography, because the pressure of the dye load may cause complete rupture of the aorta. The first treatment for aortic rupture is fluid resuscitation, usually with red blood cell products. A large-bore chest tube is inserted and placed to gravity or suction drainage, preferably with a blood salvaging device. In some patients insertion of the chest tube may provide a route for exsanguination by eliminating the tamponade effect. In some instances the chest tube may be clamped by the physician to prevent exsanguination and the patient immediately transported to the operating room for reparative surgery. Postoperatively the patient requires sedatives, antihypertensives, and antibiotics. Since bowel ischemia may occur secondary to hypotension, the patient may also require an exploratory laparotomy and bowel resection.

Patients with superior vena caval syndrome need emotional and psychologic support during the diagnosis and treatment phases. Some patients may need an artificial airway. The patient may undergo bronchoscopy for diagnosis of the tumor type, which is important in determining treatment. Diuretics and steroids are commonly ordered.

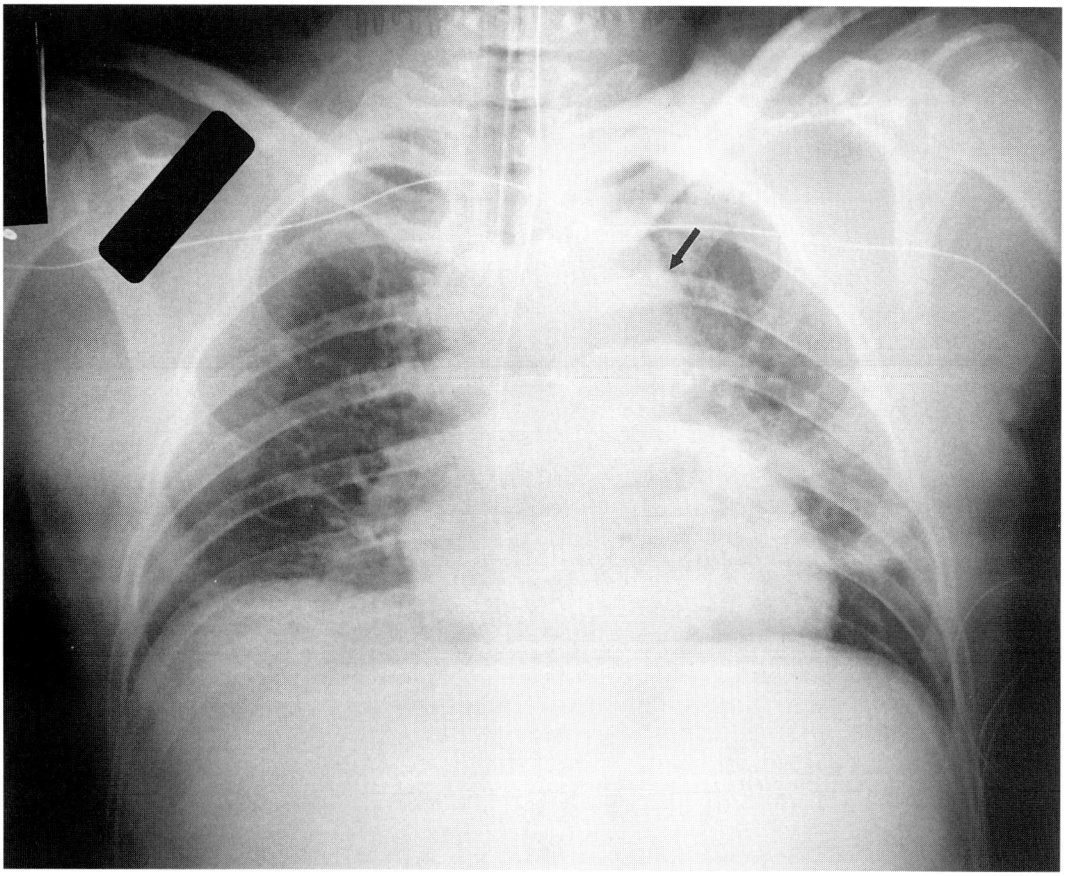

Fig. 3-47 This patient has a widened mediastinum suggestive of an aortic injury. The angiogram demonstrates a rupturing aorta that requires emergent surgical repair. Also visible are the endotracheal tube, which is too low, and a nasogastric tube.

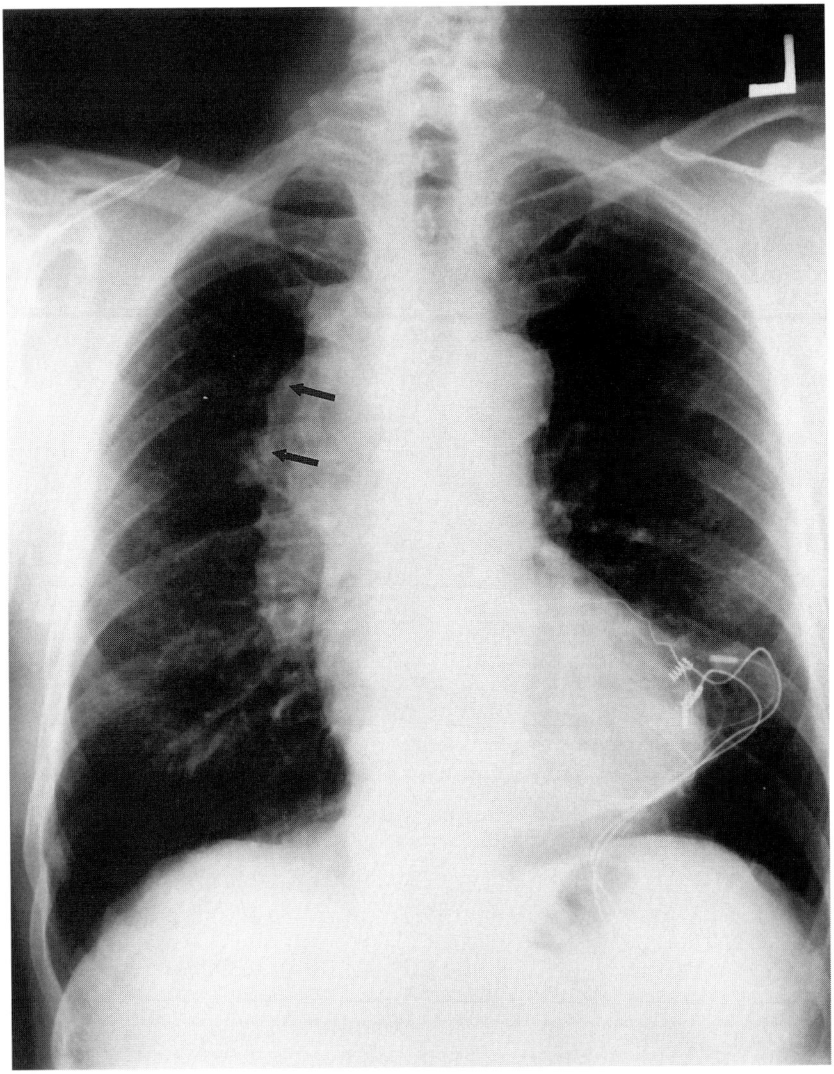

Fig. 3-48 This patient has an enlarged hilar area consistent with a right hilar tumor. Notice that the patient also has an AICD.

TEST YOURSELF

Use your knowledge of assessing a chest radiograph to answer the questions under Fig. 3-49.

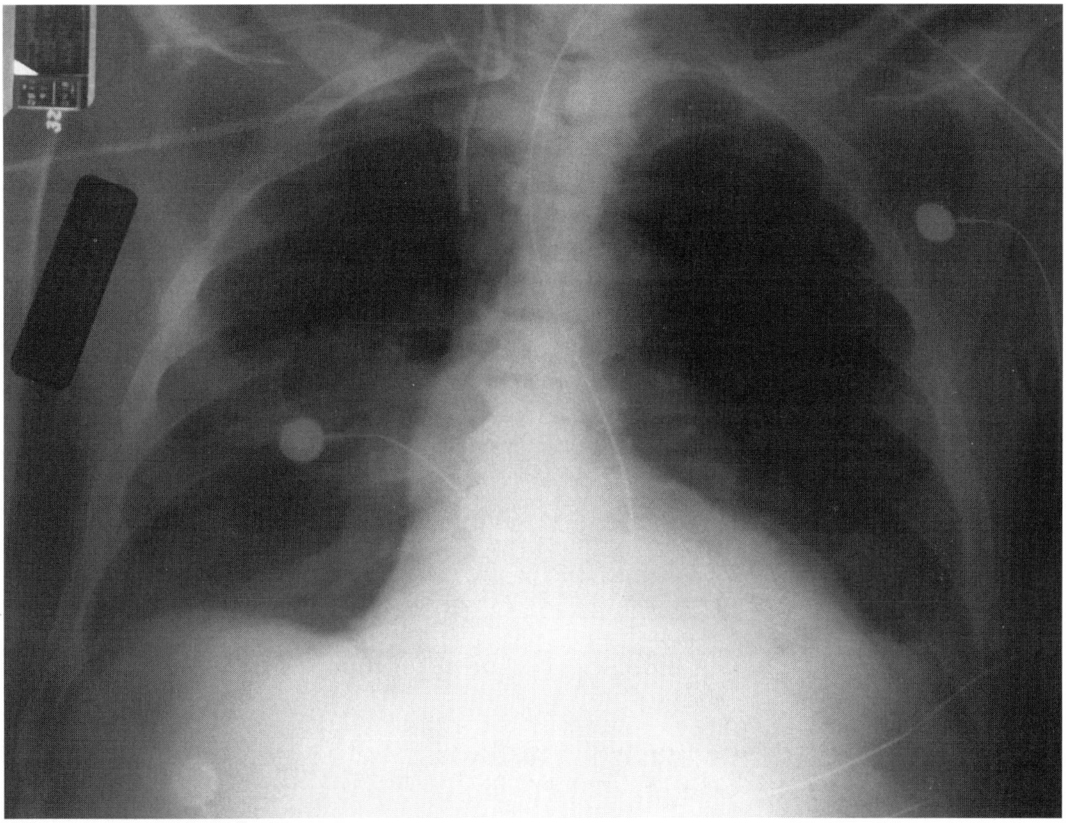

Fig. 3-49 Identify two major abnormalities visible on this chest radiograph. What is the parenchymal process? Is the catheter in good position?

BIBLIOGRAPHY

Ballinger PW: *Merrill's Atlas of radiographic positions and radiologic procedures,* ed 7, St Louis, 1991, Mosby.

Dettenmeier PA: *Pulmonary Nursing Care,* St Louis, 1992, Mosby.

Felson B, Weinstein AS, Spitz HB: *Principles of chest roentgenology: a programmed text,* Philadelphia, 1965, W.B. Saunders.

Felson B: *Chest roentgenology,* Philadelphia, 1973, W.B. Saunders.

4 Assessment of the Patient
Neurologic Radiography

The patient with neurologic dysfunction often presents a diagnostic challenge to clinicians. The signs and symptoms of a stroke may resemble those of a traumatic injury or a space-occupying lesion. Noninvasive and invasive radiographic studies are usually done quickly to diagnose the cause of the patient's deficits. The nurse who cares for patients with facial injuries, neurologic deficits, spinal cord damage, or extremity injury needs to be aware of the findings of the diagnostic x-ray exams so appropriate nursing care can be planned.

The focus of this chapter is on radiography, angiography, myelography, and nuclear medicine studies. Since 1972, the major tool for diagnosing intracranial disorders has been computed axial tomography (CAT or CT). Although an indepth discussion of CT scanning is beyond the scope of this text, it will be described where appropriate.

NORMAL STRUCTURES

The Skull

A basic understanding of the normal structures of the central nervous system that can be viewed with x-ray films is helpful in determining abnormalities. The skull is the framework of the head and is composed of eight cranial bones and fourteen facial bones. The cranium encloses the brain and protects it from external elements. The bones that make up the cranium include: the frontal, occipital, sphenoid, ethmoid, two temporal, and two parietal bones (Fig. 4-1).

The frontal bone covers the anterior of the skull and forms the forehead. Frontal sinuses (air-filled openings in the bone) are located in this bone. The

A

B

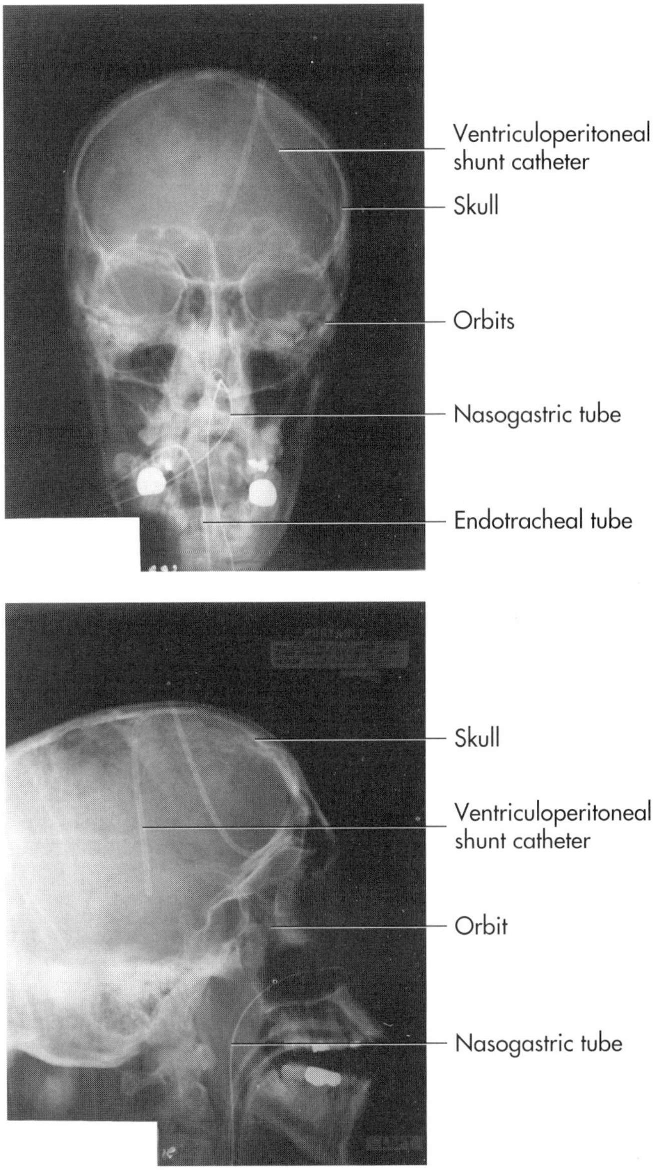

Fig. 4-1 Skull film of patient with no pathological conditions. **A,** Anterior-posterior view. **B,** Lateral view. Note: It is difficult to obtain totally normal skull radiographs because they are rarely performed with the intensive care patient unless a pathological condition is strongly suspected. This patient has an old ventricular-peritoneal shunt catheter in place. A nasogastric tube and an endotracheal tube have been inserted.

frontal lobes of the brain (the thinking, judging, word-producing area of the brain) are found immediately under the frontal bone.

The occipital bone is the large bone in the back of the skull. This bone covers the occipital lobe and contains the foramen magnum and occipital condyles, which attach the skull to the first cervical vertebra.

Under the brain on the bottom surface of the cranium is the bat wing–shaped bone called the sphenoid bone. The markings on this bone are the body, the lesser wings, the greater wings, and the sella turcica, which cradles the pituitary gland.

Hidden between the orbits of the eyes is the ethmoid bone. This bone has a perpendicular and a horizontal plate and two lateral masses. The cribriform plate, or horizontal plate, forms part of the base of the skull through which the olfactory nerve passes. The perpendicular plate is part of the nasal septum, and the lateral masses are part of the ethmoid sinuses.

The temporal bones are located at the sides and base of the cranium. These irregularly shaped bones are divided into three portions: the squamous, mastoid, and petrous portions. The squamous portion is very thin and contains the zygomatic process on its external surface. This bone is identified in traumatic injury because the middle meningeal artery runs under it on the surface of the brain. If this bone is fractured, the patient is at risk for an epidural hematoma from a tear in the middle meningeal artery.

The mastoid process is contained in the mastoid portion of the temporal bone. The mastoid bone has many foramen, or openings, to allow for the passage of blood vessels.

The petrous portion of the temporal bone is very dense and lies at the base of the skull. It contains the essential branches of the middle meningeal artery.

The parietal bones fuse at the top of the skull and cover the parietal lobes. The internal surface of these bones is concave.

The cranium has two layers, the outer table and the inner table. Between these tables is an area of cancellous bone that helps absorb blows to the skull.

In addition to these structures of the cranium, are the sutures that can be seen on skull x-ray films (Fig. 4-1). Sutures are areas in which the bones of the cranium are joined. Four sutures are visible on a radiograph: the sagittal suture in the midline joining on the top of the skull, the coronal suture connecting the frontal and parietal bones, the lambdoidal suture connecting the occipital and parietal bones, and the basilar suture or squamous suture joining the basilar surface of the occipital bone and the sphenoid bone (Marshall et al, 1990).

A normal x-ray film of the skull shows the bones that are identified on the previous page. The sutures are closed on an x-ray film of an adult. The two tables of the skull cannot be differentiated on a plain skull x-ray film (AP or lateral), but they can be seen on a CT scan.

The Brain

The brain is not visible on noninvasive x-ray films, but the cerebrum, cerebellum, and brainstem can be viewed on CT scans. Portions of these areas may also be observed with the use of arteriography.

The brain contains the cerebrum, cerebellum, and brainstem. The cerebrum is made up of two frontal, two parietal, two temporal, and one occipital lobe. The lobes of the brain lie under the bones of the cranium for which they are labeled.

The cerebellum, or "little brain," lies under the cerebrum in the posterior portion of the cranium. It is attached to the brainstem by the cerebellar peduncles. Anterior to the cerebellum in the posterior fossa are the brainstem, midbrain, pons, and medulla. Combined, the three components of the brainstem form a bridge between the spinal cord and the cerebrum. The brainstem also contains the nuclei for cranial nerves three through twelve, and the cardiac, vasomotor, and respiratory centers.

A CT scan is necessary in order to identify the cerebrum, cerebellum, and brainstem (Fig. 4-2). On a normal scan, the lobes of the brain are easily identified. In a healthy person, the brain appears gray on the CT scan and the skull appears white. Within the brain are some extremely dark areas that indicate whether they are filled with fluid. These areas include the sagittal and transverse sinuses, the ventricles, and the basal cisterns. If blood is found in brain tissue, such as when the patient has an intracerebral hemorrhage, extradural or subdural hematoma, or a cerebral contusion, the blood will appear white on the CT scan.

Covering the brain and spinal cord are the meninges; the meninges are made up of the dura mater, the arachnoid, and the pia mater. These structures protect the brain and spinal cord as well as nourish the outer surfaces. The outermost layer is the dura mater. The dura mater covers the brain, has two layers, and forms compartments by folding to support the brain. The falx cerebri descends vertically between the hemispheres (Marshall et al, 1990). The tentorium cerebelli is a tentlike fold that separates the cerebrum (the anterior and middle fossa) from the cerebellum and brainstem (the posterior fossa). The tentorium is an important anatomical landmark separating the supratentorial structures from the infratentorial structures. The falx cere-

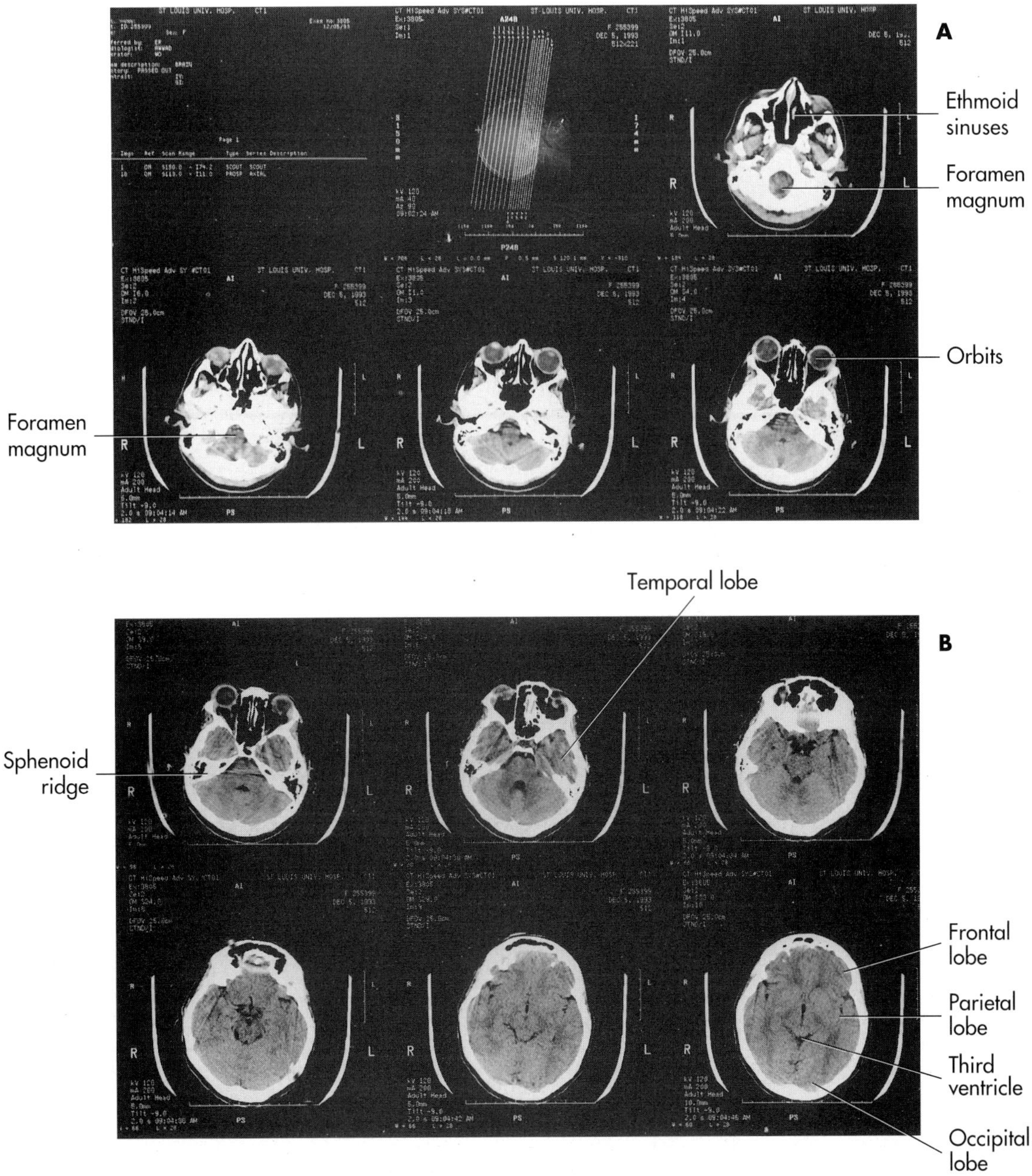

Fig. 4-2 **A** through **I,** Normal CT scan. There is no evidence of hemorrhages or tumors. Notice how the CT windows move from the top of the head down through the brain tissue. The bones of the face are easily visible in many cuts.

Continued.

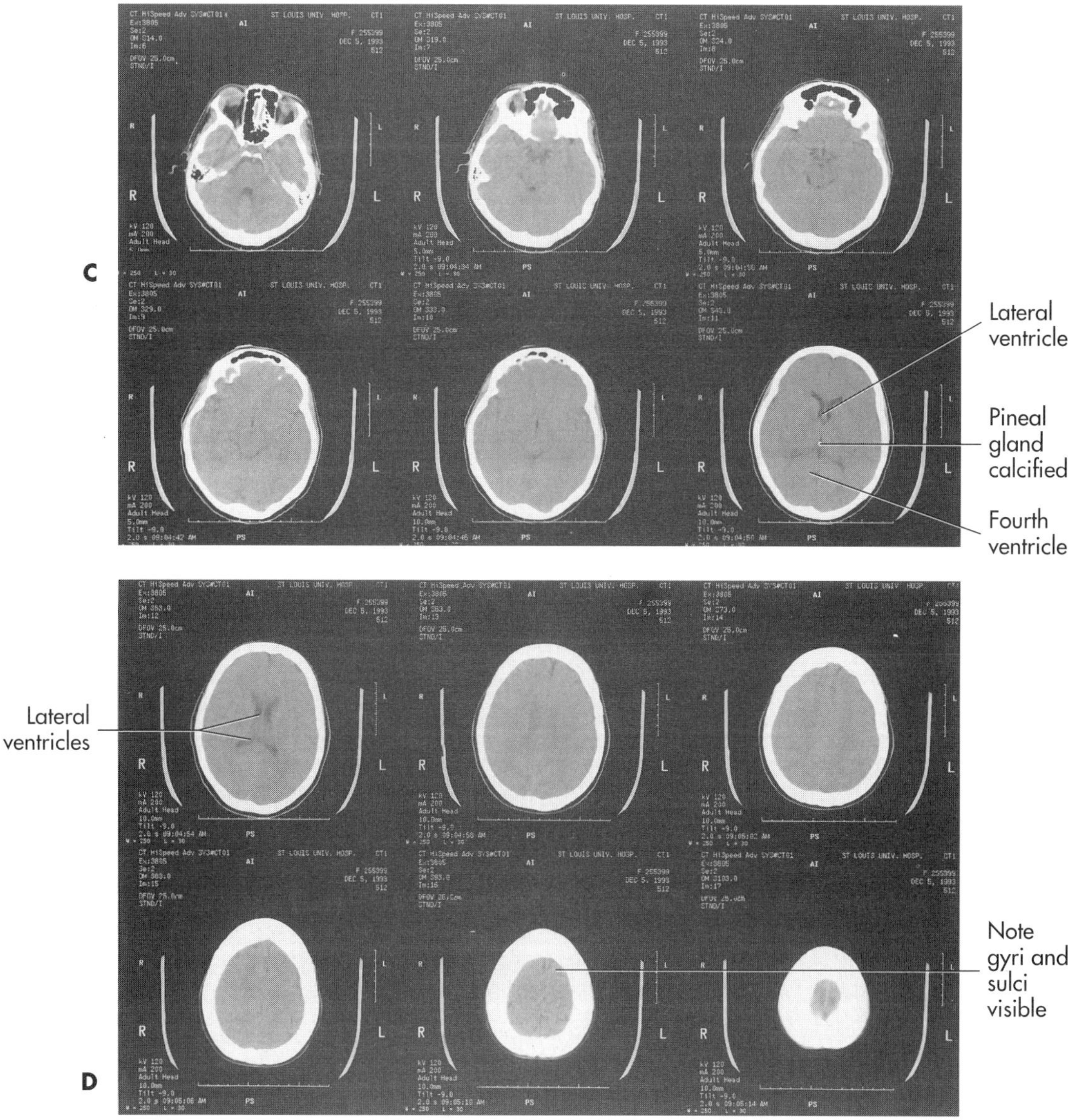
C
Lateral ventricle
Pineal gland calcified
Fourth ventricle
Lateral ventricles
Note gyri and sulci visible
D

Fig. 4-2, cont'd

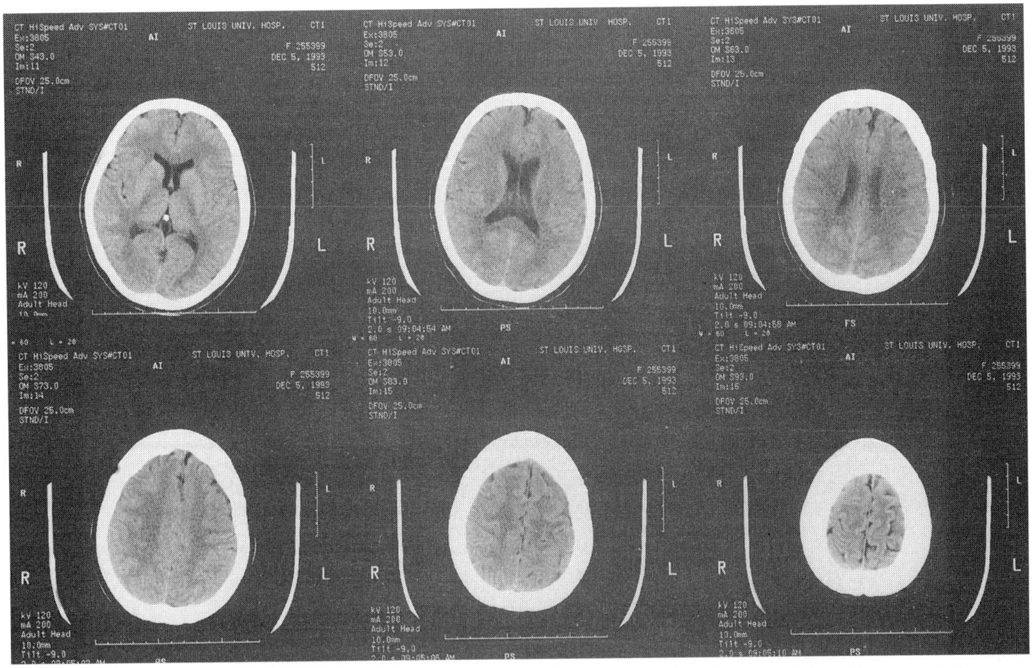

E

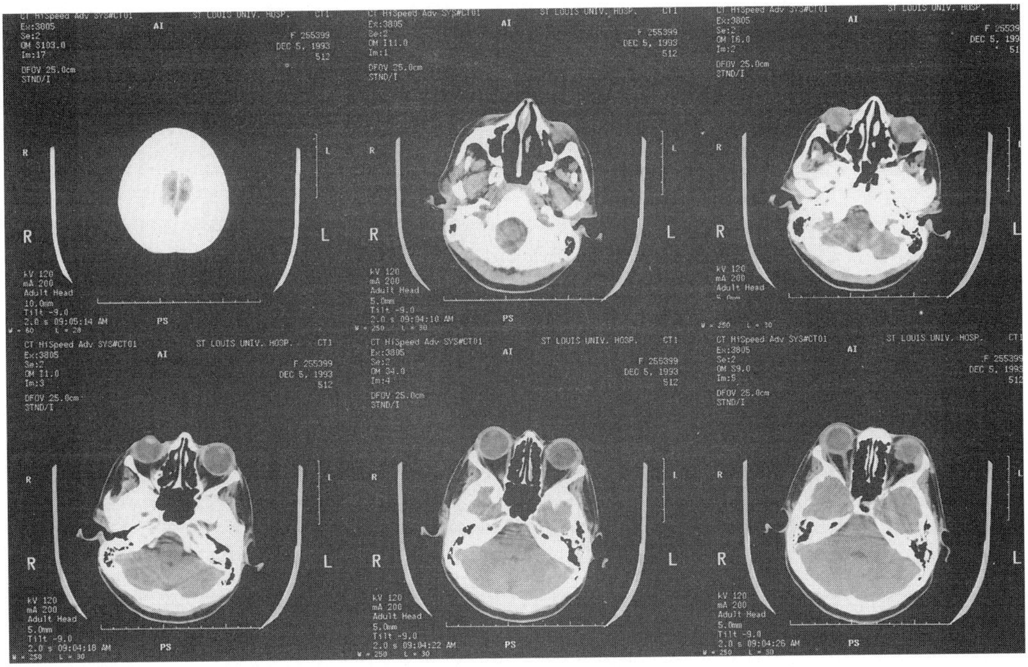

F

Fig. 4-2, cont'd

Continued.

G

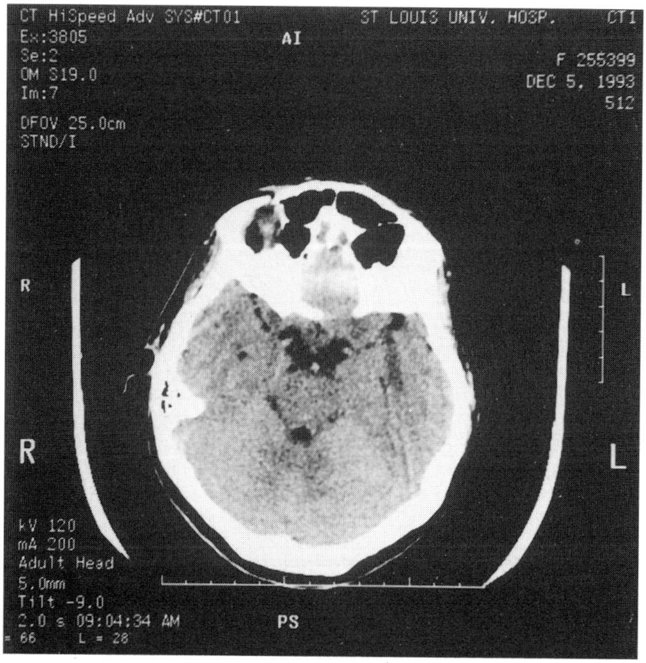

H

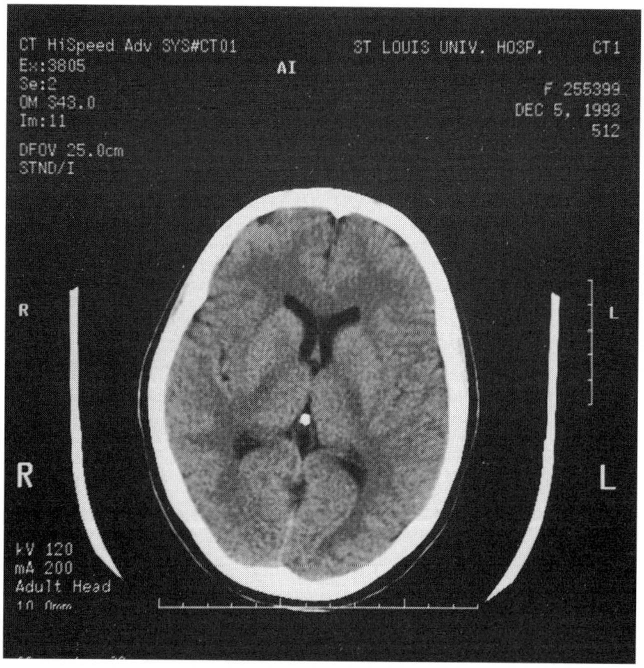

Fig. 4-2, cont'd

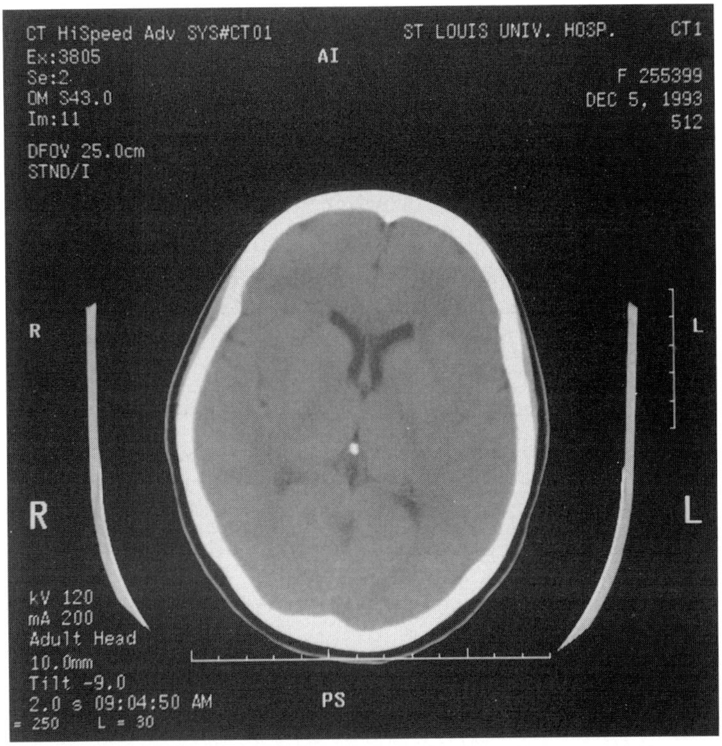
CT HiSpeed Adv SYS#CT01
ST LOUIS UNIV. HOSP.
CT1
Ex:3805
AI
Se:2
OM S43.0
Im:11
F 255399
DEC 5, 1993
512
DFOV 25.0cm
STND/I
R
L
R
L
kV 120
mA 200
Adult Head
10.0mm
Tilt -9.0
2.0 s 09:04:50 AM
= 250 L = 30
PS

Fig. 4-2, cont'd

belli separates the two lateral lobes of the cerebellum. Finally, the diaphragm sellae is the roof for the sella turcica. The spinal dura is an extension of the inner layer of the dura.

The arachnoid is the thin, filmy second layer of the meninges. Under the arachnoid is the subarachnoid space through which cerebrospinal fluid (CSF) circulates.

The pia mater is the innermost layer of the meninges. The pia mater dips into all of the grooves and sulci of the brain. In the spinal cord, the pia mater is thicker than it is in the brain.

There are some important spaces located between the skull and the brain and between the meninges to be aware of. Between the skull and the dura mater is the potential space called the epidural space. It is a potential space because it does not exist unless it is filled with something, such as blood. In the spinal cord the epidural space is between the periosteum and the dura mater. The subdural space is a narrow space that exists between the dura mater and the arachnoid. Finally there is the subarachnoid space, which was discussed earlier. A CT scan will show the dura mater, especially if it is displaced by a hematoma. The arachnoid and pia mater cannot be viewed on the CT scan.

The brain has an intricate blood supply. There is an anterior and posterior supply joined by the circle of Willis (Fig. 4-3). The anterior circulation is supplied by two internal carotid arteries. The left common carotid artery rises from the aorta; the right carotid artery rises from the innominate artery. The common carotids branch into the external and internal carotid arteries. The external carotids supply the face, and the internal carotids enter the skull and emerge under the temporal lobes. The carotid arteries give rise to the middle cerebral arteries, the anterior cerebral arteries, and the posterior communicating arteries. The two sides of the anterior supply are connected by the anterior communicating artery. The posterior circulation originates from the vertebral arteries, which come off of the subclavian arteries. The vertebral arteries enter the skull through the foramen magnum, after coming through the vertebral foramens at C5 or C6. The vertebral arteries unite at the upper medulla or lower pons to form the basilar artery. The vertebral arteries also have branches that unite and descend as the anterior spinal artery. The basilar artery is the largest artery in the posterior circulation, and it gives rise to two posterior cerebral arteries. The posterior communicating arteries connect with the posterior cerebral arteries to complete the circle. To see all of the vessels on an x-ray film, a four-vessel approach is required; that is, all four major arteries must be catheterized. The box on p. 116 lists the major arteries and their area of supply.

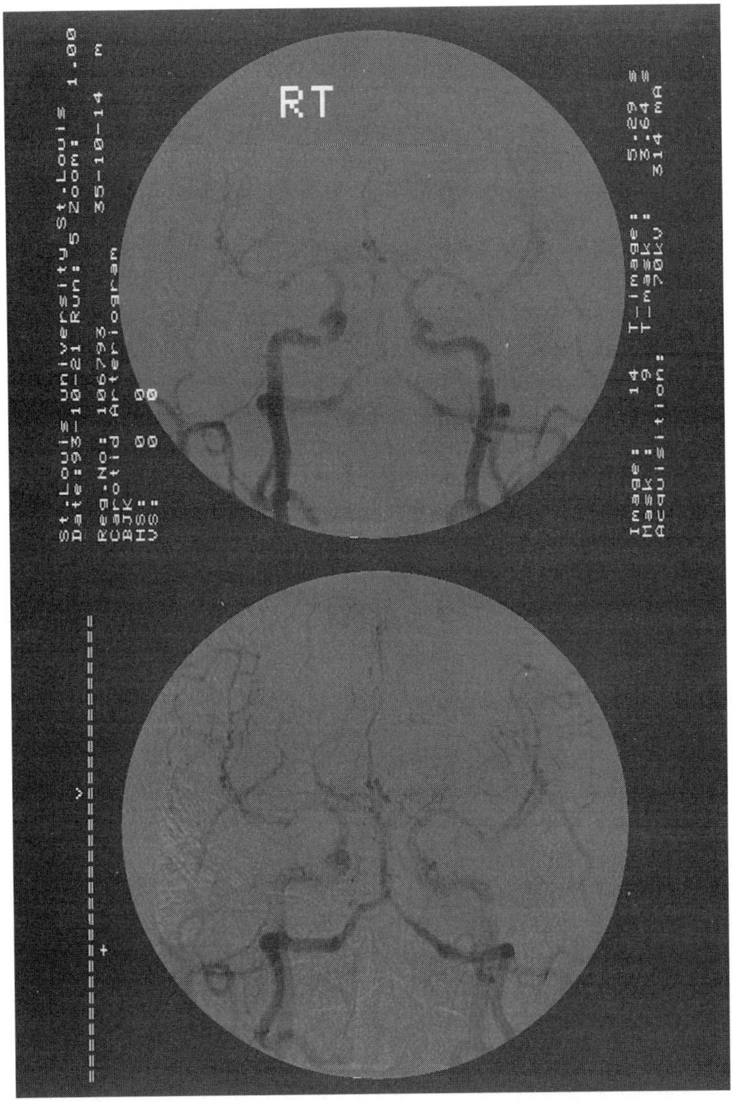

Fig. 4-3 Normal cerebral angiogram. Notice how the vessels form the circle of Willis. The upper image shows an arch injection with the anterior circulation (internal carotid) prominently displayed (i.e., darker). In the lower image the posterior circulation is darker. Notice how the two vertebral arteries join to form the basilar artery.

MAJOR ARTERIAL SUPPLY TO THE BRAIN

ANTERIOR CEREBRAL ARTERY
Inferior part of the internal capsule
Frontal lobes
Parietal lobes
Olfactory tracts
Precentral gyrus—leg area
Corpus callosum

MIDDLE CEREBRAL ARTERY
Frontal lobe—voluntary motor area*
Parietal lobe—somatosensory area*
Portion of the temporal lobe
Dura, arachnoid, pia

POSTERIOR COMMUNICATING ARTERY
Optic chiasm
Pituitary gland
Thalamus
Midbrain (upper portion)

POSTERIOR CEREBRAL ARTERY
Posterior thalamus
Visual area of occiput
Temporal lobes
Uncus

BASILAR ARTERY
Brainstem
Cerebellus

VERTEBRAL ARTERIES
Medulla
Spinal cord

*Includes speech centers.

The venous drainage of the brain can also be seen with the use of angiography. The venous system in the brain is also unique in that it is managed by dural sinuses. These sinuses are valveless (Adams and Victor, 1981). Cerebral veins drain into the sinuses, which in turn empty into the jugular veins.

On the angiogram the arterial circulation as described above can be observed. The dye fills the entire circulation, anterior and posterior. It also shows the smaller branches that rise from the circle of Willis. On the lateral view, it is possible to view one hemisphere's flow, including the medial meningeal artery. During the venous phase of the angiogram the sagittal and transverse sinuses and the vein of Galen can be identified. The venous system is identical in all persons, thus any displacement of these vessels indicates a space-occupying lesion.

The ventricular system is another system that nourishes the brain and spinal cord. The two lateral ventricles (the third and the fourth) produce and store CSF. The lateral ventricles are deep between the hemispheres, with the frontal horns between the frontal lobes, the parietal horns in the parietal lobes, the occipital horns in the occipital lobe, and the temporal horns between the temporal lobes. The CSF circulates around the brain and spinal cord. A blockage to this circulation or the inability to absorb the CSF into the sinuses will cause hydrocephalus, which appears as a dilatation of the ventricles.

The Vertebral Column

The vertebral column is the bony protection of the spinal cord that provides support to the head and trunk. The spine is composed of 33 vertebrae: 7 cervical, 12 thoracic, 5 lumbar, 5 sacral (fused), and 4 coccygeal (fused). A typical vertebrae includes the body, pedicle, laminae, and spinous process. Only the first and second cervical vertebrae (the atlas and the axis respectively), look different. The vertebrae are held in appropriate alignment by several ligaments, including the anterior and posterior ligaments and the ligament flava, which connects the lamina of adjacent vertebrae. The vertebral column is S-shaped (convex in the cervical and lumbar areas and concave in the thoracic area). The vertebral column can be easily viewed on an x-ray film.

Each vertebrae can be seen on AP and lateral films. The entire spine can be viewed including the cervical, thoracic, lumbar, and sacral sections (Figs. 4-4 and 4-5). Fractures in the vertebral body, laminae, pedicles, and spinous process can easily be identified. Vertebrae that are displaced from their normal position can also be seen. Tomograms are usually ordered following a lateral or AP x-ray film if any question of a fracture or displacement remains.

CT scanning is useful to further define abnormalities in the vertebral column, especially small, hairline fractures or disruptions of the nerve roots.

One component of the vertebral column that is critical to normal functioning is the intervertebral disc. The disc is the fibrocartilage between each vertebra that functions as a shock absorber to cushion movements. The disc has a central core of gelatin-like material, called the *nucleus pulposa*, that is surrounded by a fibrous capsule, called the *annulus fibrosa*.

The Spinal Cord

The spinal cord runs through the central canal of the vertebral column. It is continuous with the brain and is part of the central nervous system. Extending from the upper border of the first cervical vertebra, the cord ends

A

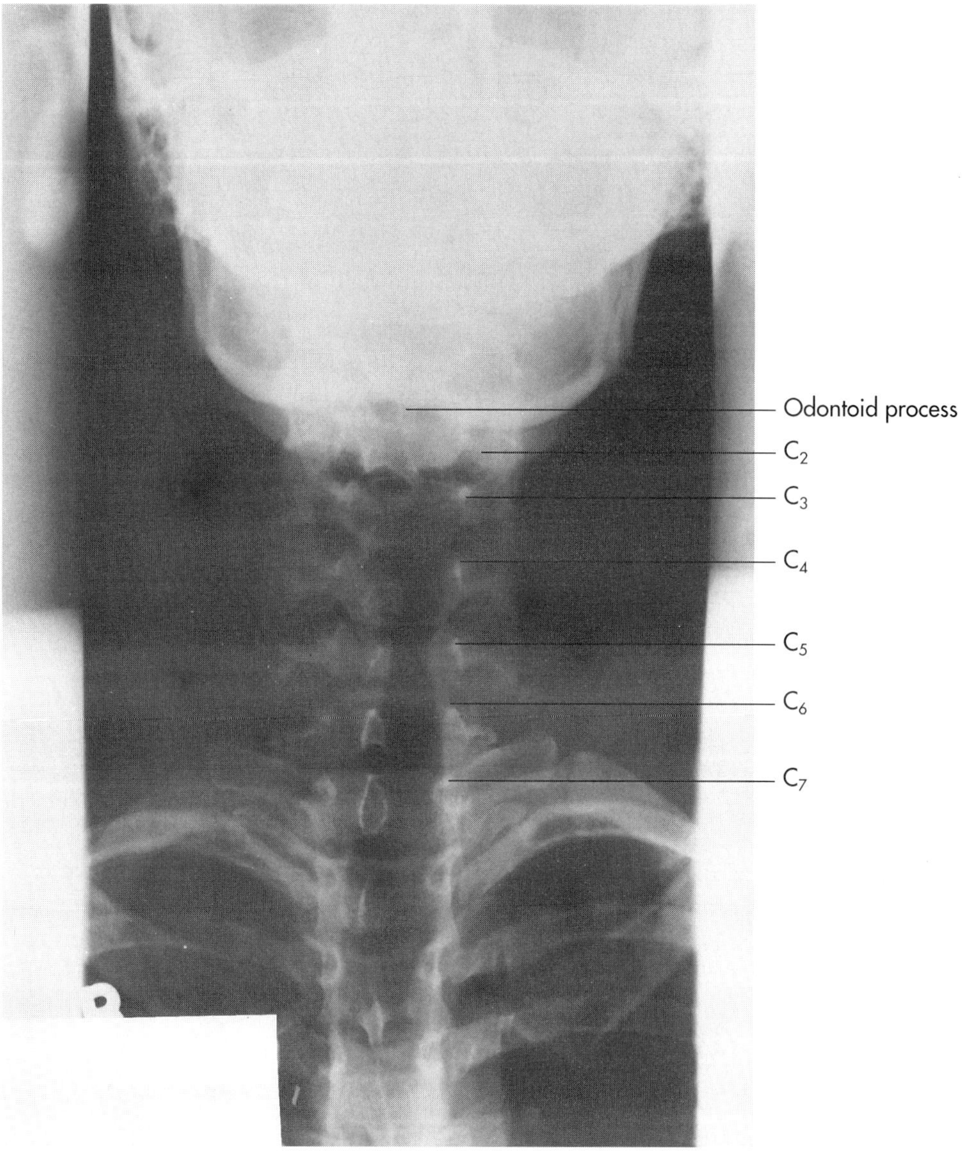

Fig. 4-4 Normal cervical spine radiograph. **A,** Anterior-posterior view. Notice how the vertebral bodies are evenly spaced and aligned.

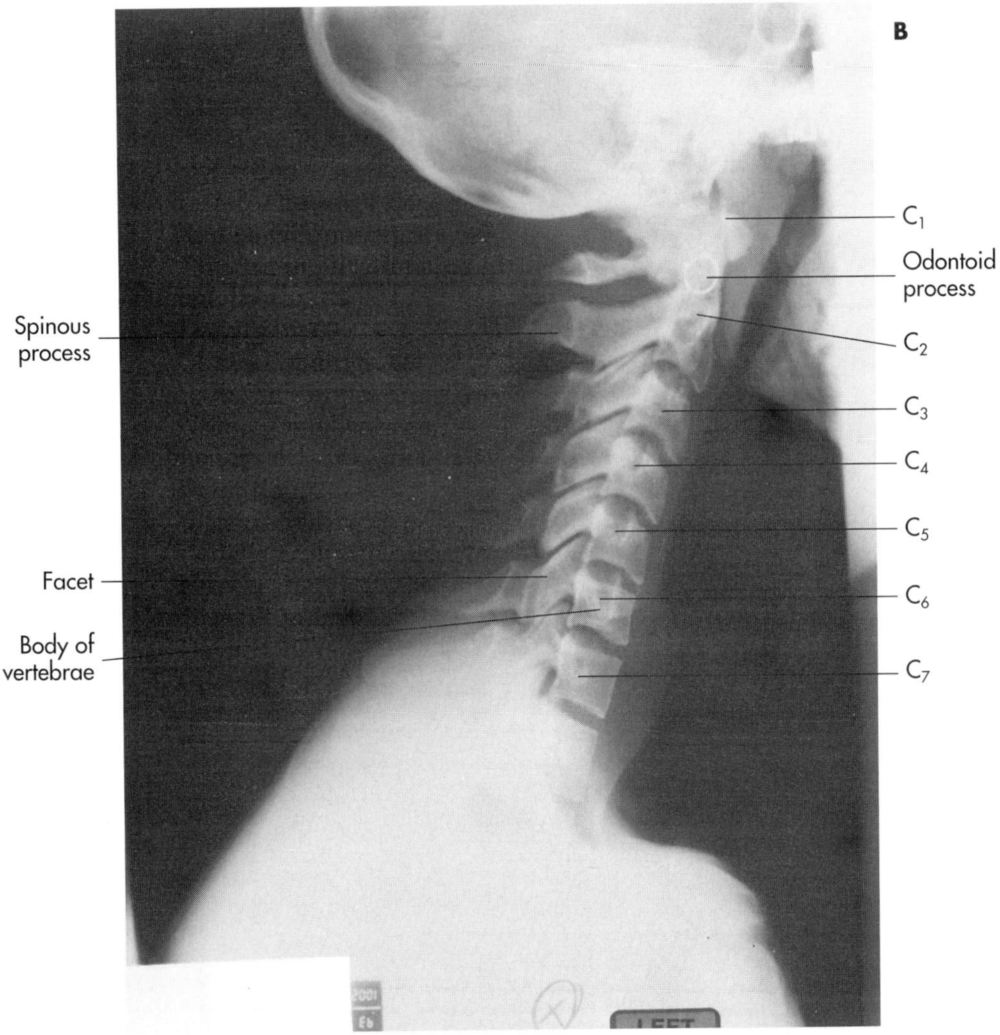

Fig. 4-4, cont'd. Normal cervical spine radiograph. **B,** Lateral view. Notice how the vertebral bodies are evenly spaced and aligned.

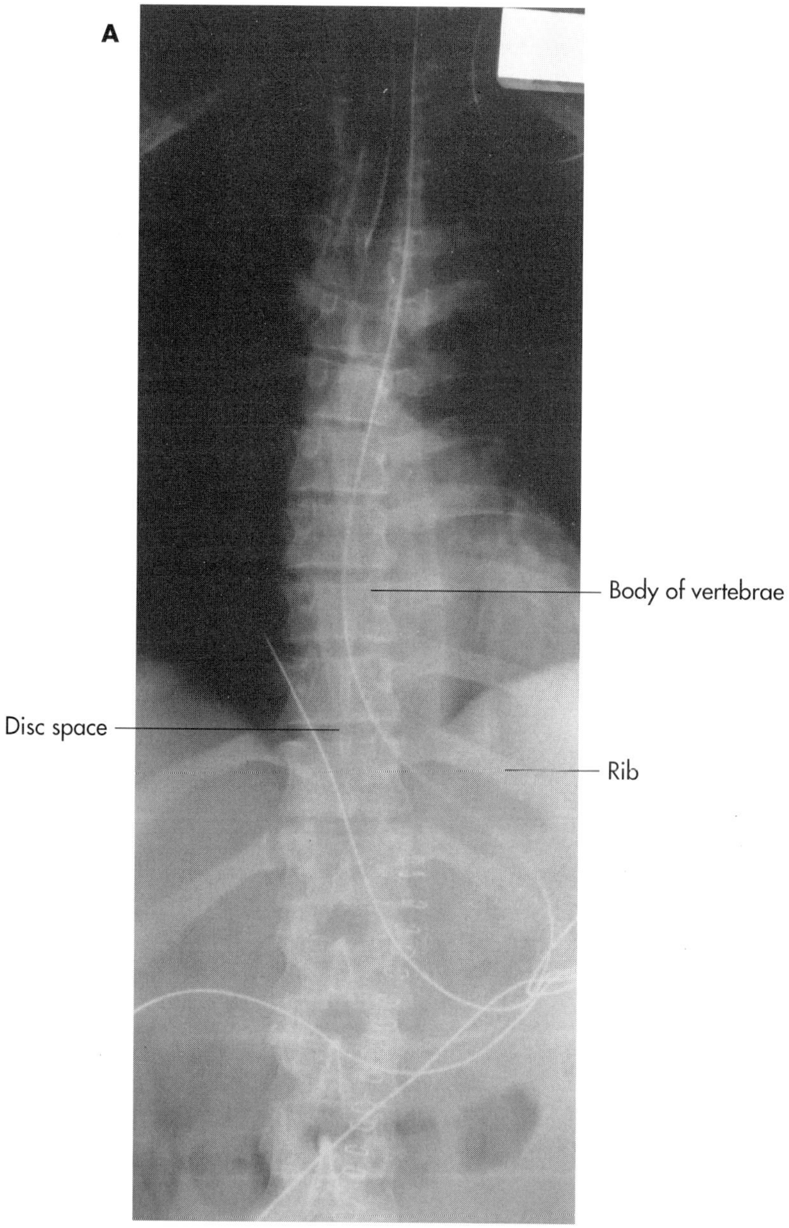

Fig. 4-5 **A** and **B,** Normal anterior-posterior and lateral radiograph of the thoracolumbar area of the spine. Notice how the vertebral bodies are evenly spaced and aligned.

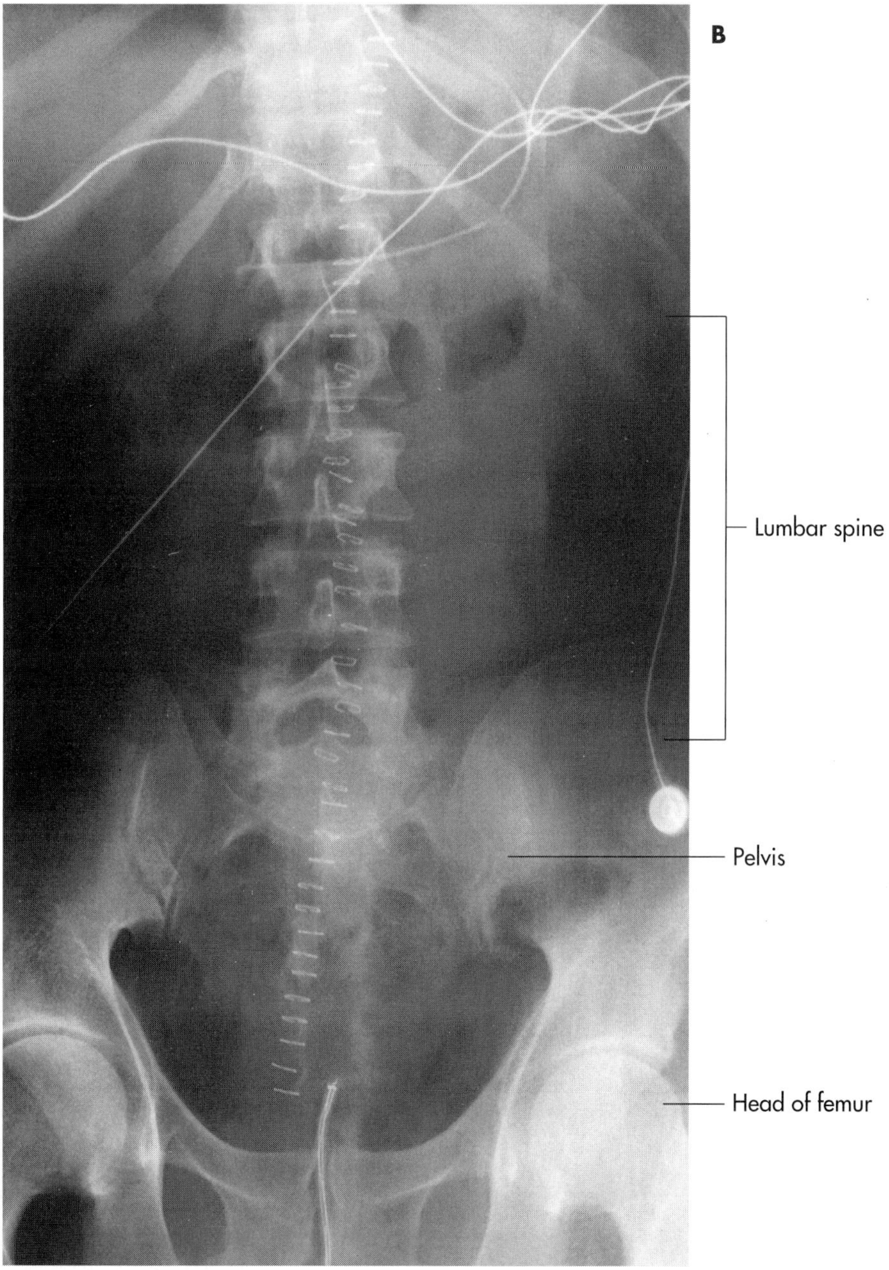
B
Lumbar spine
Pelvis
Head of femur

Fig. 4-5, cont'd

at the level of the second lumbar vertebra in adults. Below this level, the spinal roots collect to form the conus medullaris.

The 31 pairs of spinal nerves exit from the spinal cord. There are 8 cervical, 12 thoracic, 5 lumbar, 5 sacral, and 1 coccygeal nerve. Each spinal nerve has a dorsal root, which is sensory, and an anterior or ventral root, which is motor.

The spinal cord is composed of gray and white matter. The gray matter is in the shape of an H. The anterior horn of the gray matter contains the motor cells; the posterior horns contain the sensory cells. Interconnecting neurons are contained in the middle of the gray matter. The white matter tracts transmit information up and down the spinal cord (Table 4-1). Table 4-2 shows the areas of motor control by nerve root.

Table 4-1 Major white matter tracts

Name	Origin	End point	Function
Posterior columns	Spinal cord	Cerebellar and basal ganglia	Sensory pathways for muscle, joint sensation, vibration, and position sense
Spinocerebellar tracts	Spinal cord	Cerebellum	Information from muscles of extremities and trunk for coordinated movement
Spinothalamic tracts	Spinal cord	Thalamus	
Ventral			Impulses of touch
Lateral			Pain and temperature sensation
Corticospinal	Cerebral cortex of frontal lobe	Spine	Originate on the motor cortex to control contralateral motor movement for voluntary motor response

Table 4-2 Motor innervation

Spinal nerves	Muscles
C-1 to C-4	Neck (flexion, lateral flexion, extension, rotation)
C-3 to C-5	Diaphragm (respirations)
C-5 to C-6	Shoulder movement and flexion of elbow
C-5 to C-7	Forward thrust of shoulder
C-5 to C-8	Adduction of arm from front to back
C-6 to C-8	Extension of forearm and wrist
C-7, C-8, T-1	Flexion of wrist
T-1 to T-12	Control of thoracic, abdominal, and back muscles
L-1 to L-3	Flexion of hip
L-2 to L-4	Extension of leg and adduction of thigh
L-4, L-5, S-1, S-2	Abduction of thigh and flexion of lower leg
L-4 to L-5	Dorsal flexion of foot
L-5, S-1, S-2	Plantar flexion of foot
S-2, S-3, S-4	Perineal area and sphincters

A plain x-ray film does not show the disc or the spinal cord; it shows the space between the vertebrae (not the disc). Narrowing of the space between the vertebrae may indicate a problem with the disc. A CT scan is necessary to see the disc and spinal cord. With a CT scan, the spinal cord can be viewed, but gray and white matter cannot. Neurologic radiographic abnormalities follow.

Bleeding into the skull

INTRACEREBRAL HEMORRHAGE

Definition

Intracerebral hemorrhage, also known as hemorrhagic stroke, is caused by bleeding into the brain tissue from a rupture of one of the arteries in the brain. The hemorrhage is usually related to hypertension or trauma. This is the most devastating form of stroke and is associated with a high rate of mortality and morbidity.

Clinical Findings

Patient assessment generally shows systemic hypertension and a slow heart rate. Neurologic changes are related to the area of the brain affected by the hemorrhage. Symptoms may include a decreased level of consciousness, pupillary changes, contralateral hemiparesis or hemiplegia, or coma.

Radiologic Appearance

Two tests are generally performed to diagnose intracerebral bleeding: the CT scan and the cerebral angiogram. The initial CT scan may show hyperdense areas where hemorrhage is present (Fig. 4-6). Depending on when the bleeding occurred, the brain tissue surrounding the hemorrhage may be swollen. Several days after the hemorrhage, the area, if not resected, becomes isodense, then hypodense. The angiogram may show the vessels that bled or the cause of the hemorrhage, such as an aneurysm or an arteriovenous malformation.

Nursing Implications

The patient may need to be sedated for the CT scan because any movement will distort the reading of the scan. The patient must be positioned lying flat, which may cause increased intracranial pressure or worsen neurologic symptoms. For the extremely restless patient, a head strap may be used to hold the head still.

The patient should be sedated before a cerebral angiogram. Again, the patient must lie flat. Close monitoring is necessary throughout the test.

The patient must be monitored carefully after the test, especially his or her blood pressure because antihypertensive therapy may be required. The head of the bed should be elevated to 30 degrees following the diagnostic study. Frequent neurologic assessments are necessary, especially for the first 72 hours following the hemorrhage. Intracranial pressure monitoring may be necessary.

INTRACRANIAL EPIDURAL HEMATOMA

Definition

Epidural hematoma is a result of bleeding into the potential space between the inner table of the skull and the dura. Epidural hematomas account for

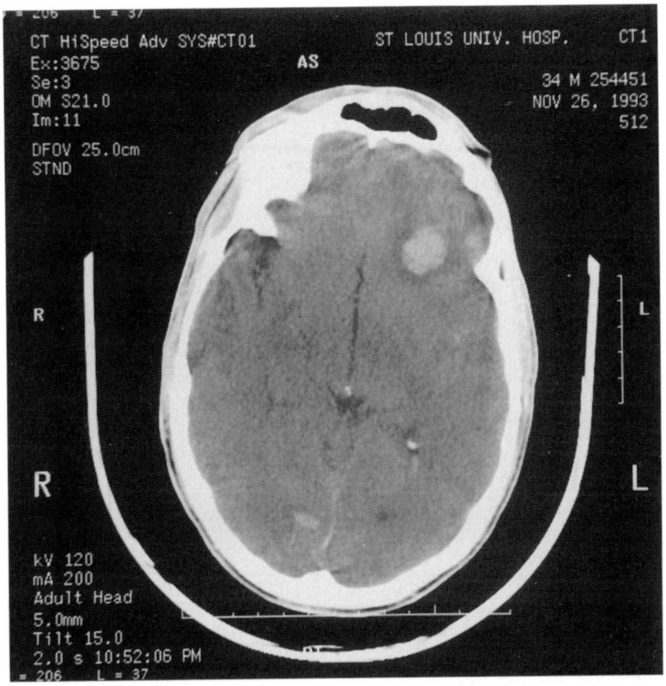

A

Fig. 4-6 **A** through **C,** Intracerebral bleeding—hemorrhagic stroke. Notice the hyperdense area in the left frontal lobe, and surrounding edema. The CT scan shows a mild mass effect on the ventricles because they are smaller.

Continued.

B

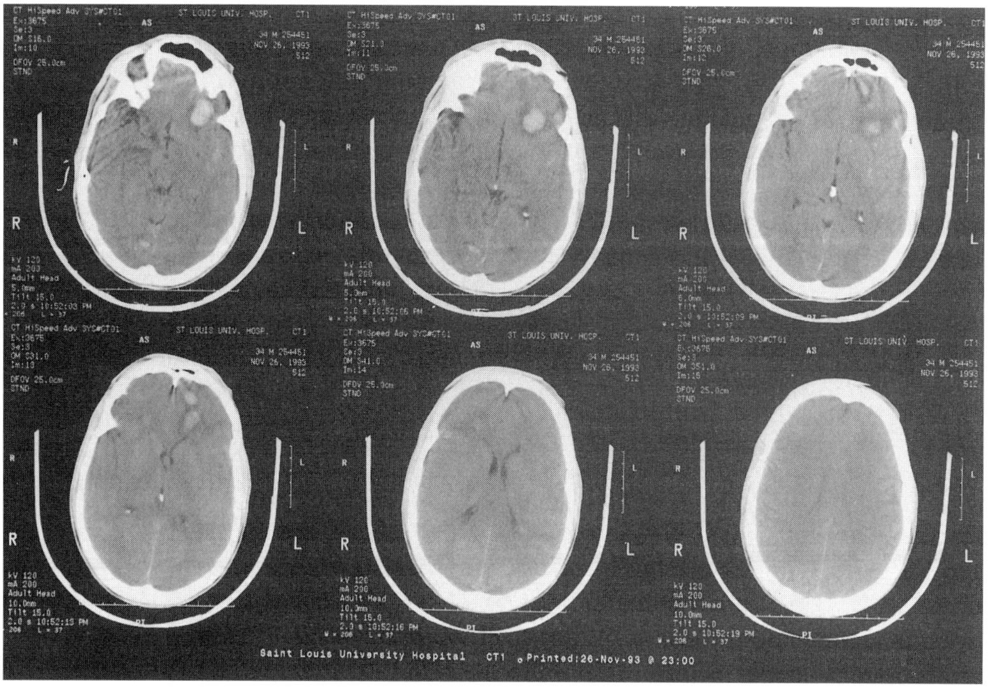

C

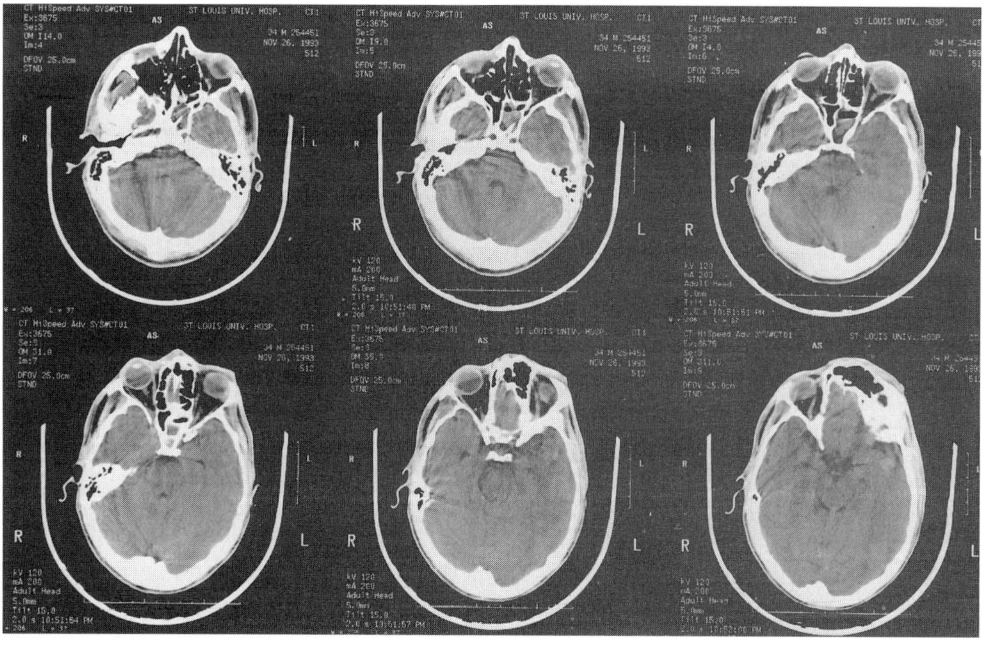

Fig. 4-6, cont'd

2% of all head injuries. The middle meningeal artery generally causes the bleeding.

Clinical Findings

The patient usually has a history of moderate to severe head trauma with a skull fracture. The patient may have exhibited the classic triad of symptoms: unconsciousness at the time of the accident, a period of alertness, then a rapid deterioration in consciousness. As the hematoma enlarges, the patient will demonstrate signs of central herniation. The patient will have a unilateral, fixed, dilated pupil on the side of the hematoma, a contralateral hemiparesis, and a loss of consciousness. The patient may also have Cushing's syndrome: a rising systolic blood pressure, a widening pulse pressure, and bradycardia. The patient may have flexor or extensor posturing.

Radiologic Appearance

In approximately 85% of these patients, a fracture of the squamous portion of the temporal bone can be seen on a lateral skull radiograph. A CT scan may or may not be necessary. If a CT scan is performed, the hematoma will appear as a hyperdense area immediately beneath the skull, pushing the dura mater away from the skull and compressing the brain (Fig. 4-7).

Nursing Implications

The lateral skull radiograph may be taken in the emergency department while the patient is lying on a stretcher. If a CT scan is necessary, the patient must lie flat during the scan, which may worsen the neurologic status. The patient requires rapid surgical evacuation to prevent neurologic devastation.

INTRACRANIAL SUBARACHNOID HEMORRHAGE

Definition

Subarachnoid hemorrhage can occur as a result of a rupture of a cerebral aneurysm (most common), subdural bleeding, or the spread of intraventricular blood into the subarachnoid space. Lumbar puncture was formerly performed before CT scanning and showed hemorrhagic spinal fluid in all tubes. A subarachnoid hemorrhage was diagnosed but the cause was not known.

A

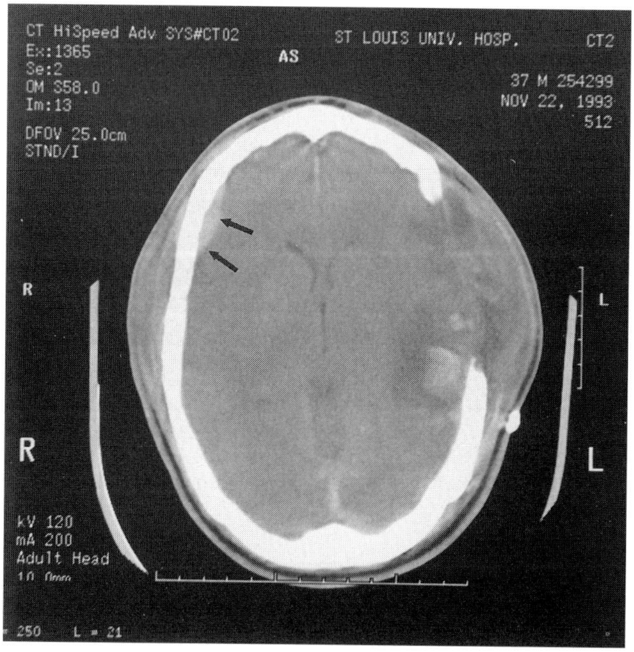

B

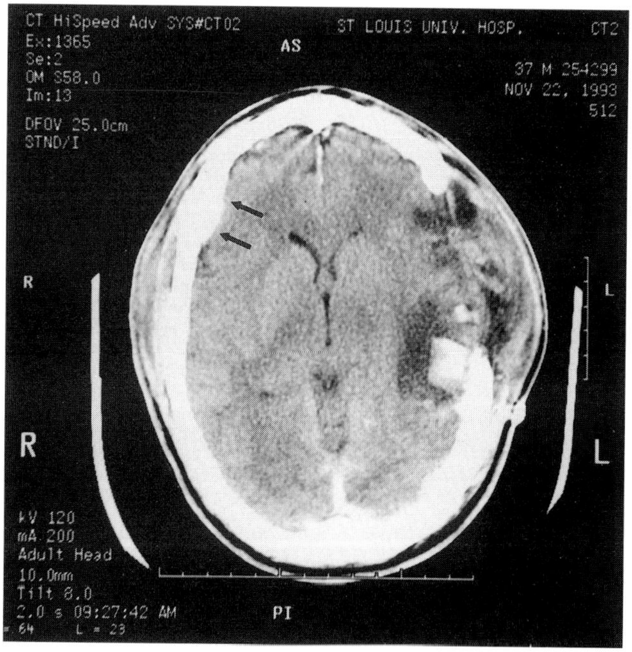

Fig. 4-7 **A** through **E,** Epidural intracranial hemorrhage. Notice the biconvex hyperdense extra-axial blood collection; this is consistent with an epidural hemorrhage in the right frontal region. Note that this patient has had a portion of the skull removed (to evacuate an expanding subdural hematoma). There is significant soft-tissue swelling.

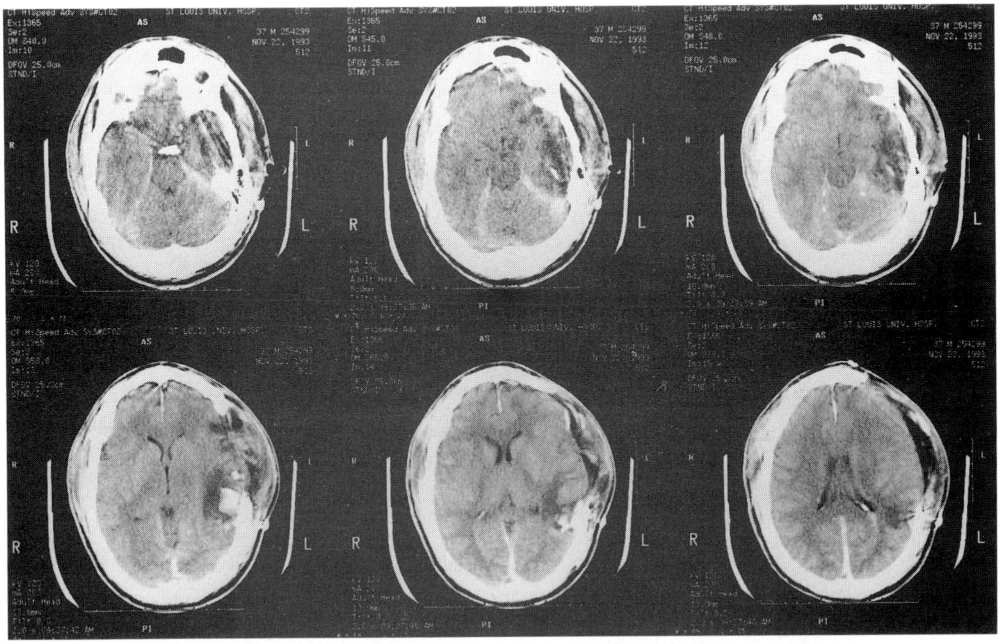

C

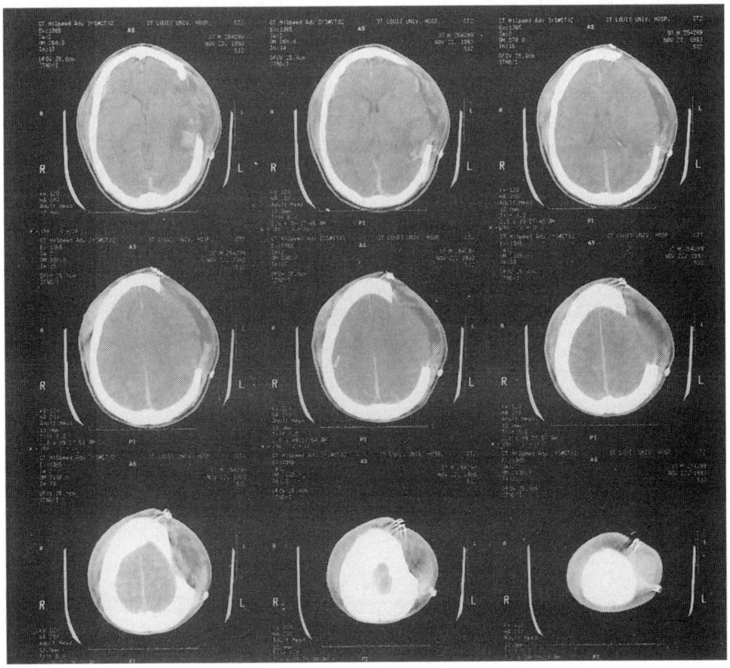

D

Fig. 4-7, cont'd

Continued.

E

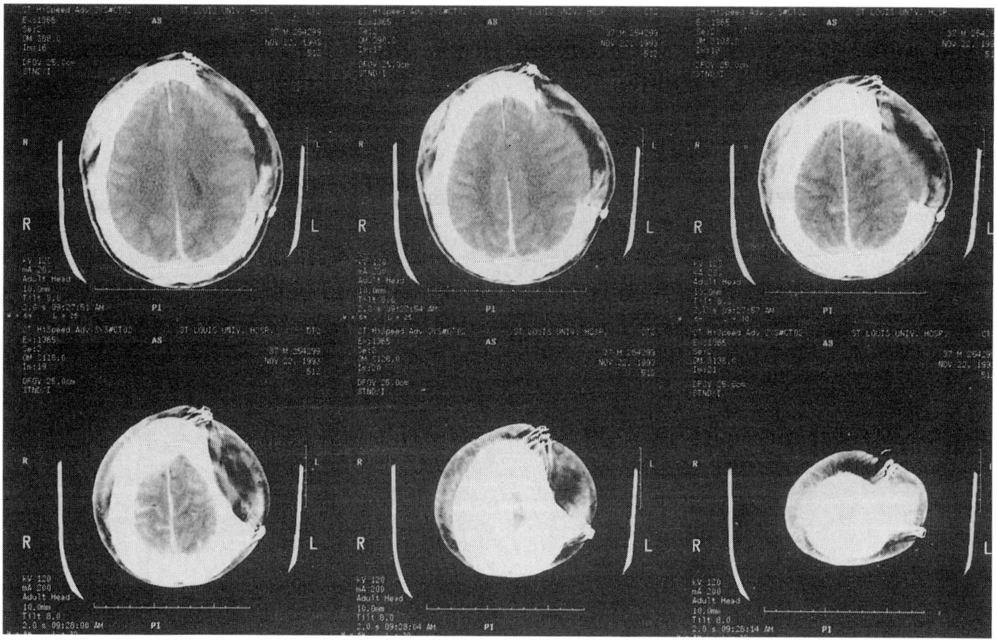

Fig. 4-7, cont'd

The bleeding is often diagnosed by CT scan, but angiography is needed to determine the vessel that has caused the bleeding. Aneurysms are classified by shape and etiology (Table 4-3). They usually occur at bifurcations of the large arteries at the base of the brain. Most (85% of) aneurysms develop in the anterior circulation. Cerebral vasospasm is the leading cause of morbidity and mortality.

Table 4-3

Aneurysm	Features
Berry	Most common; has a neck or stem
Saccular	Any aneurysm with a saccular outpouching
Fusiform	An outpouching on an artery without a neck
Traumatic	Results from traumatic injury to a blood vessel
Mycotic	Rare; caused by a septic emboli
Charcot-Bouchard	Microscopic aneurysm associated with hypertension Usually in basal ganglia and brainstem
Dissecting	Blood is forced between the intimal and medial layer of the vessel, caused by trauma atherosclerosis or inflammation

Clinical Findings

The patient will have a rapid onset of severe headache, photophobia, and a stiff neck. Depending on the cause of the subarachnoid bleeding, the patient may have a decreased level of consciousness and some cranial nerve involvement. If the patient has vasospasm, the severity of neurologic symptoms will increase.

Radiologic Appearance

A CT scan is performed without contrast material initially to establish the extent and location of the subarachnoid bleeding. This initial scan can also be useful in the early diagnosis of the potential for vasospasm. The area that includes the vasospastic vessels will show areas of ischemia and hypodensity on the scan (Fig. 4-8). A later CT scan with contrast media should be per-

A

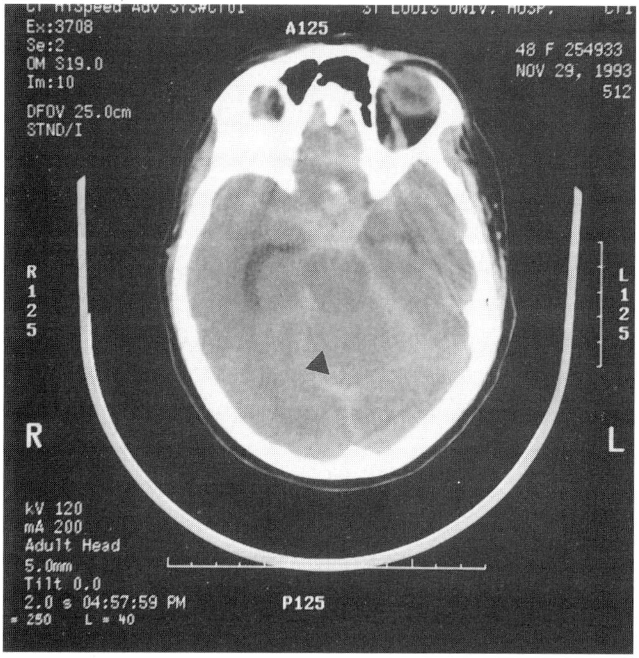

B

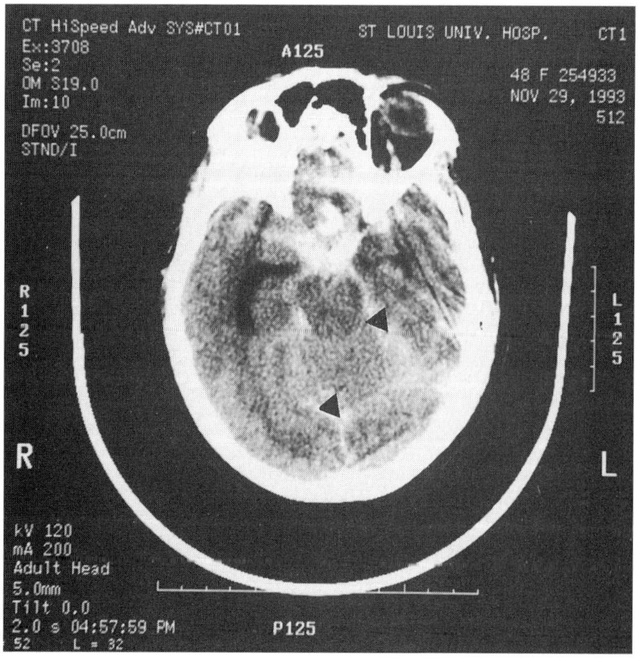

Fig. 4-8 **A** through **F,** Subarachnoid intracranial bleeding—subarachnoid hemorrhage. In this brain window there is acute hemorrhage in the subarachnoid space. The hyperdense regions are demarcated. Acute bleeding appears white in color.

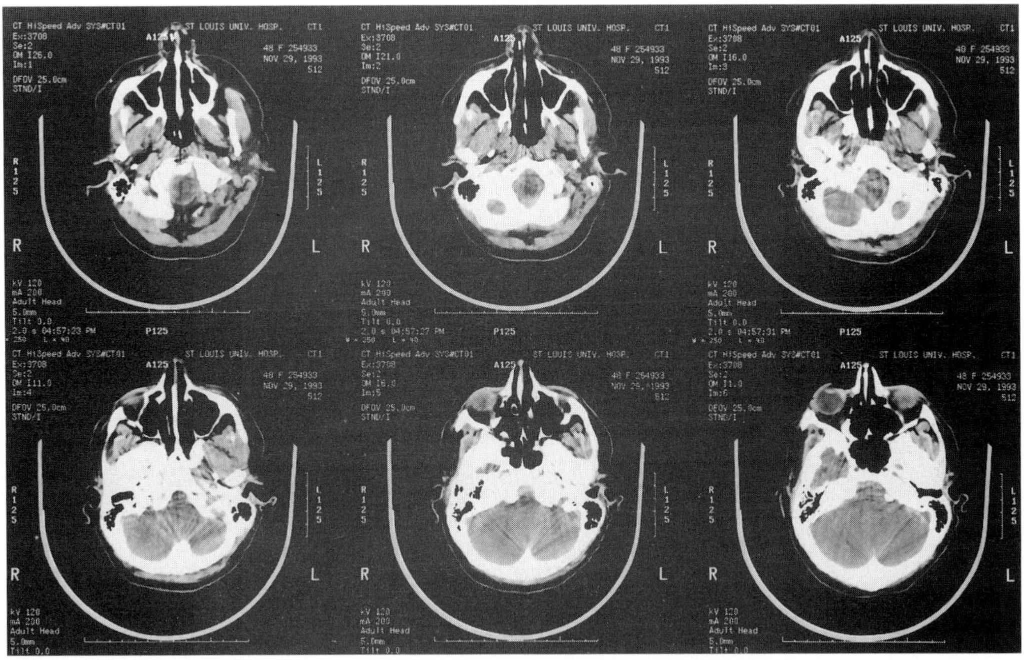

C

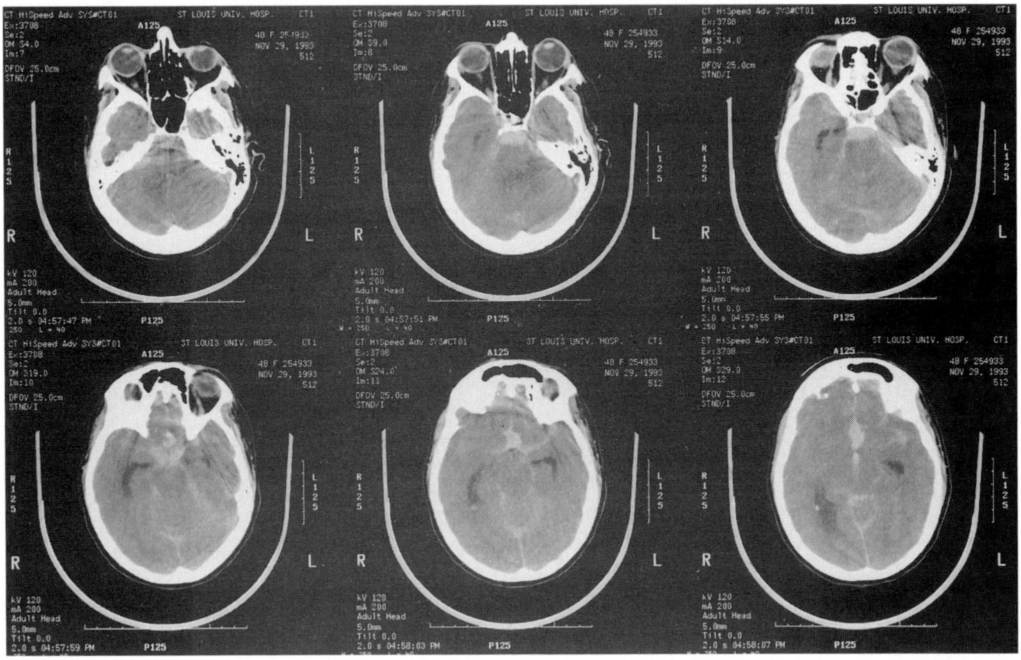

D

Fig. 4-8, cont'd.

Continued.

E

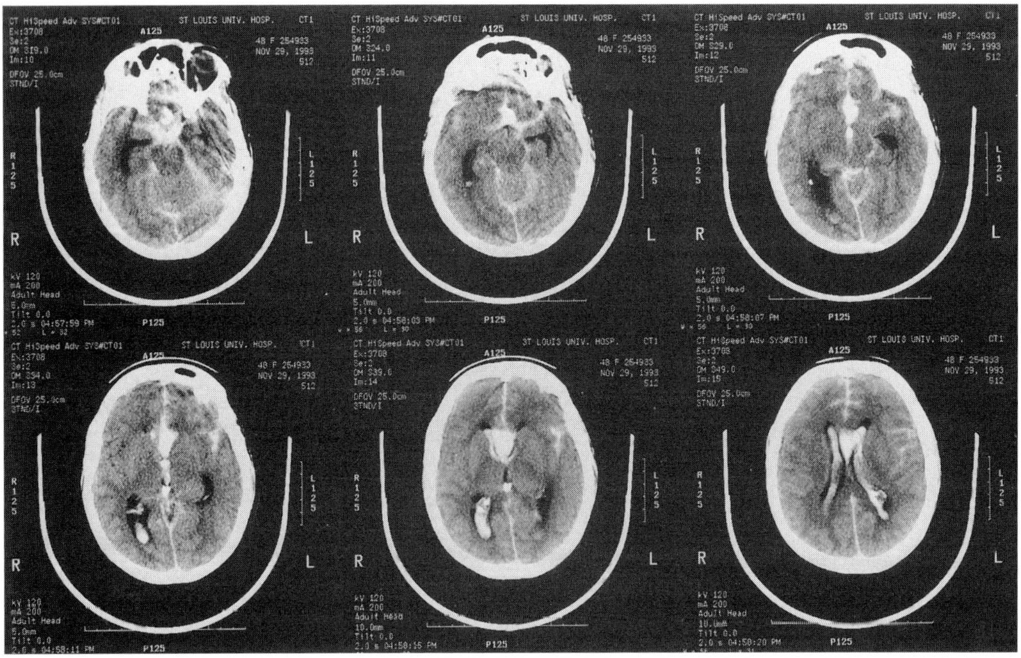

F

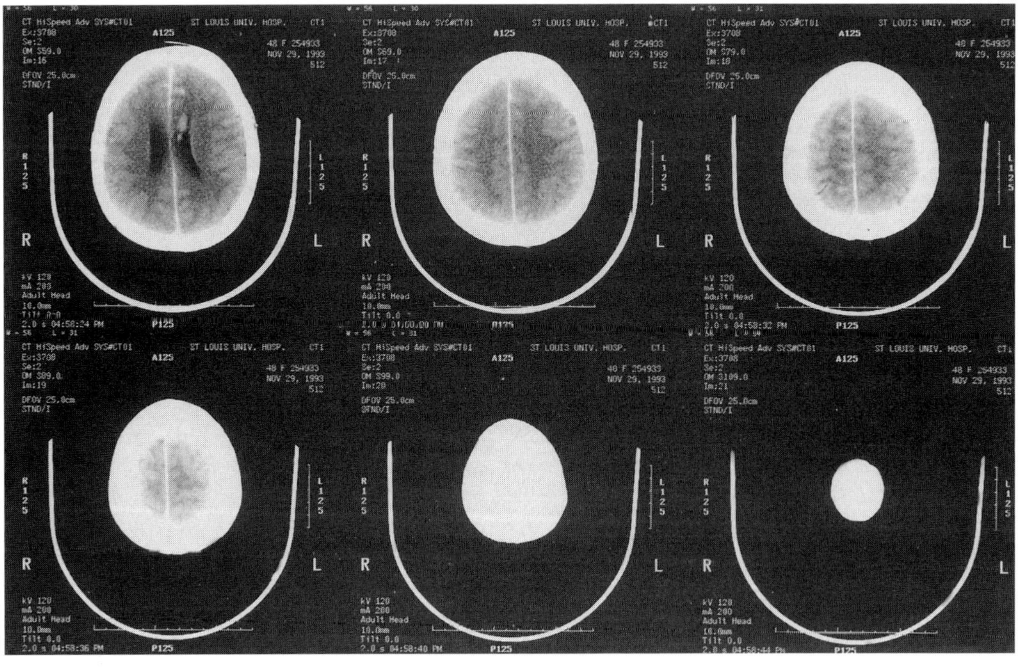

Fig. 4-8, cont'd

formed about 72 hours after the initial hemorrhage. This second CT scan may be used to locate the area of the aneurysm or arteriovenous malformation. The CT scan performed at this time may also show hydrocephalus from blood clogging the arachnoid villi.

Cerebral angiography is the best diagnostic tool for an aneurysm or other vascular malformation that may have caused the subarachnoid bleeding. Fig. 4-9 shows a cerebral angiogram that pinpoints the location of the aneurysm. The aneurysm that has ruptured will look different from one that has not. The ruptured aneurysm will have a small hyperdense area called a "tit" where a clot has formed to seal the rupture. Viewing the entire cerebral circulation during the angiogram is important to identify the actual number of aneurysms that may be present, although usually only one ruptures and bleeds. Very small aneurysms may obliterate themselves when they bleed and may not be found on angiogram. Following surgical repair of the aneurysm by clipping, an intraoperative angiogram may be performed to ensure obliteration of the aneurysmal sac and the integrity of the parent artery. An angiogram should also be performed before the patient's discharge.

Nursing Implications

The patient may need to be sedated and kept in a dark, quiet environment before the aneurysm is clipped. Control of blood pressure is critical to prevent another hemorrhage, but the blood pressure must be maintained at a level high enough to prevent ischemia. Close monitoring and frequent neurologic assessment are also very important.

INTRACRANIAL SUBDURAL HEMATOMA

Definition

A hemorrhage into the subdural space is generally caused by trauma. The bleeding is usually venous and is caused by stretching and tearing of the bridging veins of the dura mater. A subdural hematoma is found in 10% to 15% of all patients with head injuries. The bleeding may progress into the subarachnoid space.

A

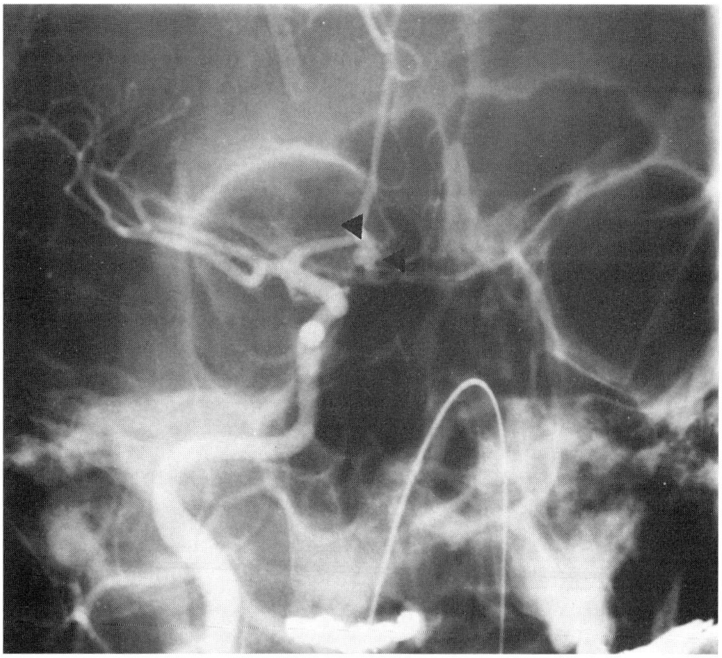

B

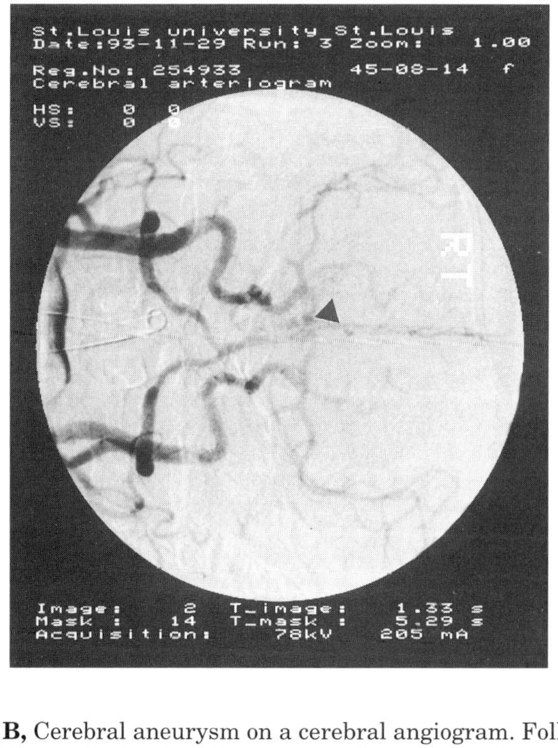

Fig. 4-9 **A** and **B,** Cerebral aneurysm on a cerebral angiogram. Follow the internal carotid to the middle cerebral artery. The arrow points out an abnormal sac-like structure an anterior communicating artery aneurysm.

Clinical Findings

The patient usually has a history of trauma. Generally some loss of consciousness has occurred at the time of the accident. The patient will have a rapid onset of neurologic dysfunction in the case of an acute subdural hematoma including coma, hemiplegia, and pupillary changes. If the injury happened more than 48 hours before the onset of symptoms, the patient may have a subacute subdural hematoma. In this case the patient will have a more subtle onset of symptoms, which are often mistaken for signs of increased intracranial pressure.

Radiologic Appearance

An x-ray film is generally not helpful in diagnosing a subdural hemorrhage, except in the case of a chronic subdural hemorrhage, which may be calcified. The CT scan will demonstrate a hyperdense area usually over the surface of the brain, convex in shape, and pushing the brain away from the skull (Fig. 4-10).

Nursing Implications

The patient must lie flat for a CT scan, which may increase intracranial pressure and worsen the patient's symptoms. For an acute subdural hematoma, immediate surgical evacuation of the clot is necessary. Continuous neurologic assessment and monitoring is necessary to detect any deterioration in neurologic function.

Blood flow studies

CEREBROVASCULAR ACCIDENT

Definition

Cerebrovascular accident (stroke) is the third most common cause of death in the United States. It is the most common cause of neurologic disability in adults. Stroke is a syndrome characterized by the gradual or rapid onset of neurologic deficits that last for 24 hours or more (Adams and Victor, 1981).

A

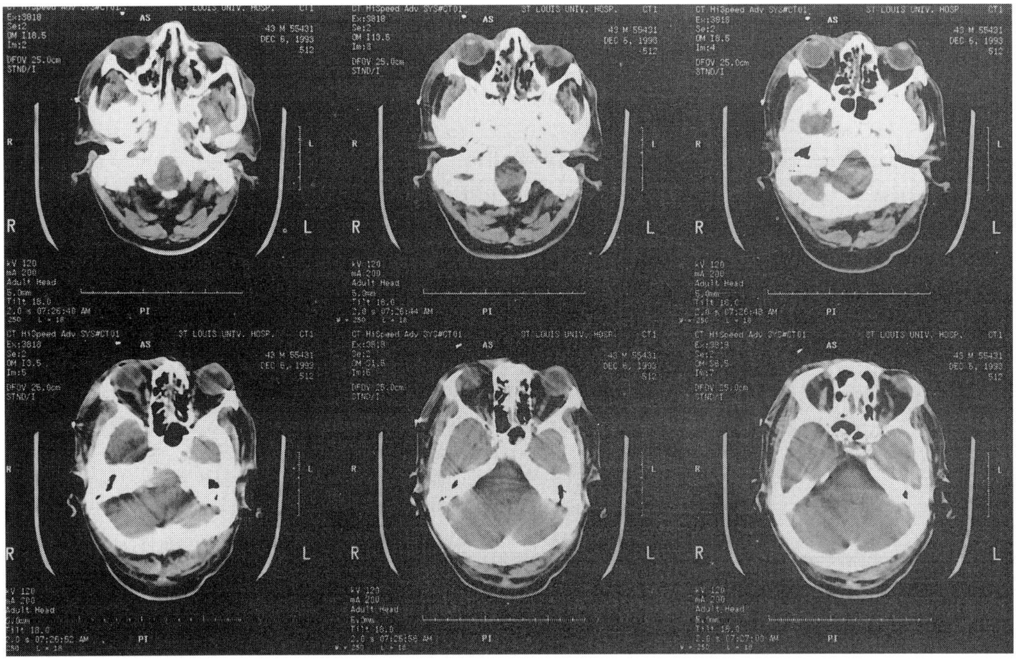

B

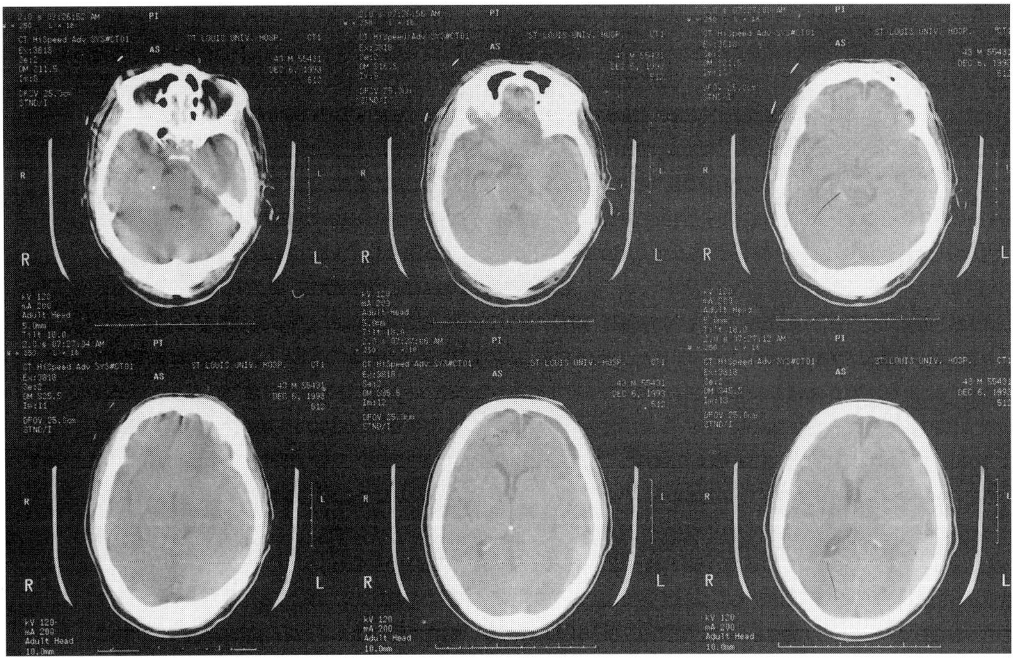

Fig. 4-10 **A** through **F,** Subdural intracranial hemorrhage. This patient has an extraaxial (out of brain) hyperdense blood collection in the subdural space. There is a mass effect, as seen by the ventricles being pushed to the right of the midline.

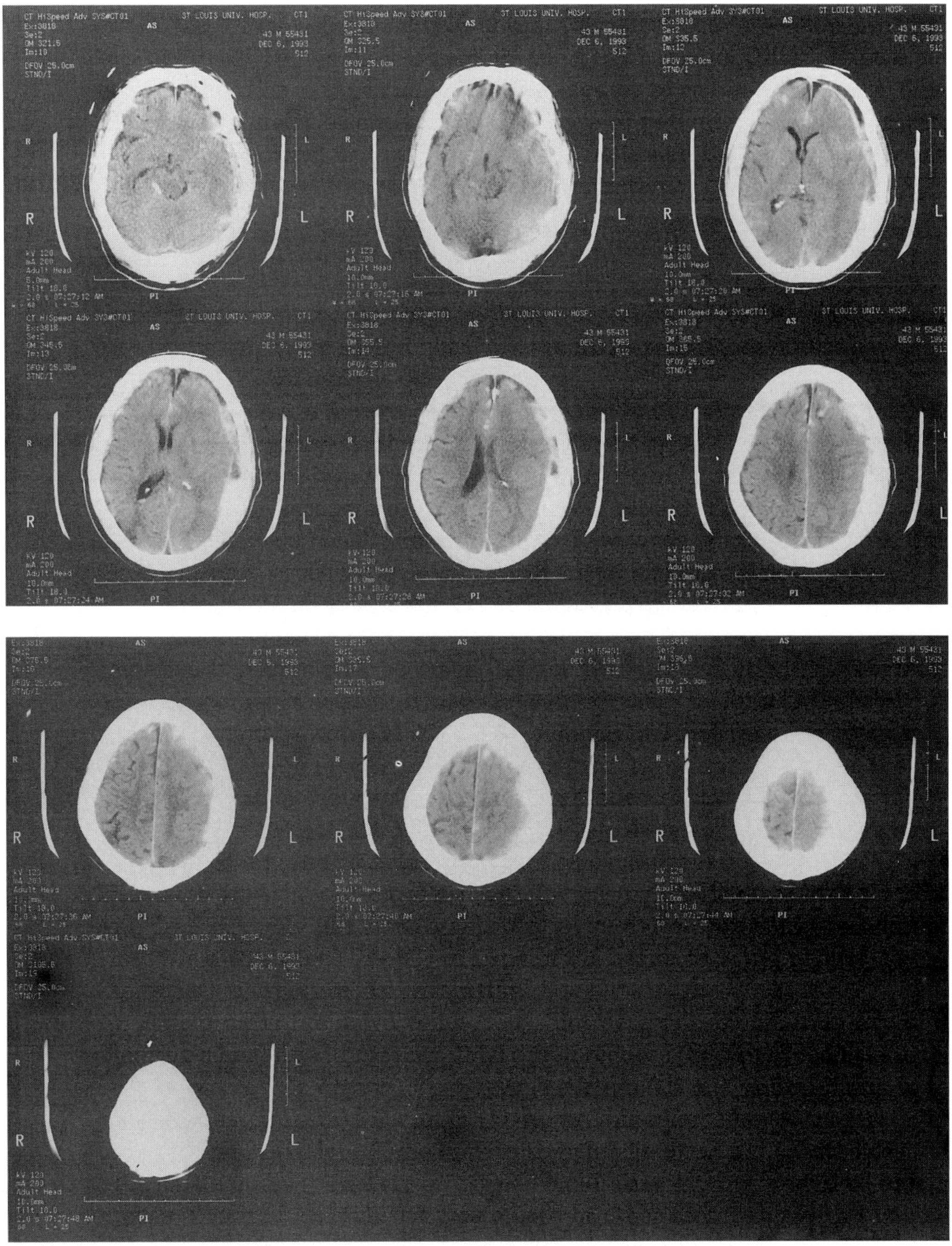

C

D

Fig. 4-10, cont'd

Continued.

E
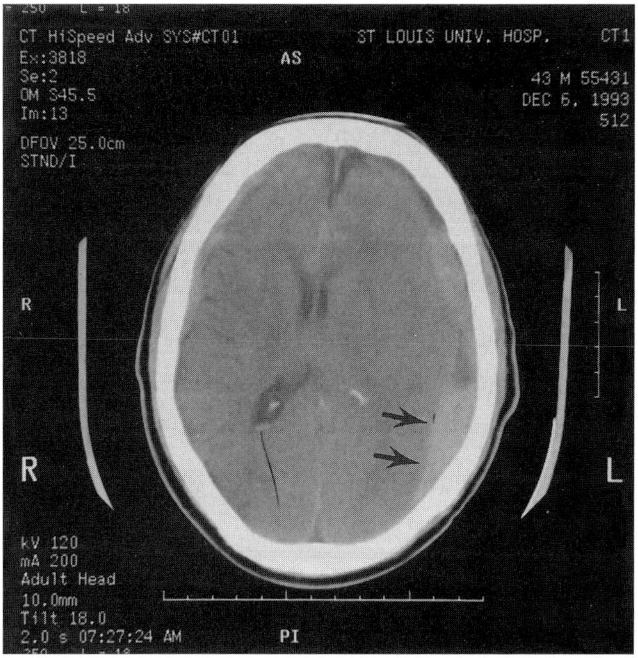

F
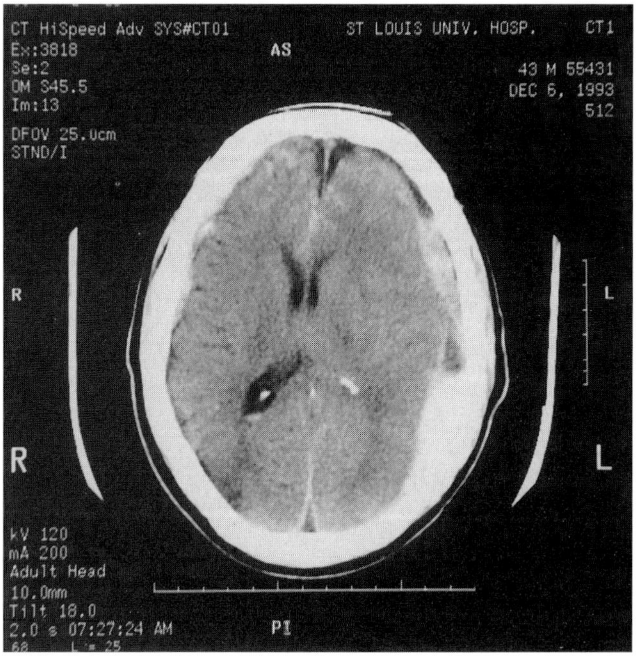

Fig. 4-10, cont'd

The deficits follow a specific vascular supply. The two major categories of stroke are ischemic and hemorrhagic strokes. In this section, the focus will be on diagnosing ischemic stroke.

Ischemic stroke is divided into two categories based on the mechanism of ischemia: thrombotic and embolic ischemia. Thrombotic stroke involves the anterior circulation five times more frequently than the vertebrobasilar distribution. This mechanism of stroke is related to atherosclerosis. The patient typically has warnings prior to the completed stroke, including transient ischemic attacks (TIAs) and reversible ischemic neurologic deficits (RINDs). The onset of symptoms is gradual.

Embolic ischemic stroke tends to occur in younger patients. The onset of symptoms is rapid once the emboli occludes a major cerebral vessel. The left middle cerebral artery is most commonly affected by an embolic phenomenon (Marshall et al, 1990).

Clinical Findings

The patient will generally arrive at the hospital with hypertension and variable neurologic deficits that depend on the areas affected by the ischemia. With thrombotic stroke, onset of symptoms will be gradual; with an embolic phenomenon onset of symptoms is sudden.

Radiologic Appearance

Cerebral angiography is the diagnostic test of choice for cerebrovascular accidents. A cerebral angiogram consists of injecting a radiopaque dye into an artery to view the extracranial and intracranial blood vessels. The approach is either by direct insertion into the carotid arteries or by catheterization through the femoral or brachial artery to the carotid and vertebral arteries. Radiographs are then taken at various intervals after the injection (Fig. 4-11).

Digital subtraction angiography is a computer-assisted radiographic procedure for viewing the cerebral vessels. The image produced is made more distinct by eliminating other anatomical structures using the computer. Images are recorded before and after the injection of the contrast medium and the first image is subtracted from the second (Marshall et al, 1990).

Study of the aortic arch in a patient with suspected thrombotic stroke is important because the common carotid arteries may also have atherosclerosis, which will require an endarterectomy. These studies are more commonly performed if the patient has presented with TIAs and RINDs.

Nursing Implications

For both types of angiograms the patient is allowed nothing to eat or drink for about 6 hours prior to the test. The patient is usually sedated before the angiogram. After the procedure, the patient needs complete bed rest for about 8 hours. Fluids should be forced to 3000 ml over a 24-hour period.

The patient is positioned flat for both a CT scan and an angiogram. This position may worsen the neurologic symptoms. Continued neurologic assessment is extremely important to determine the extent of the neurologic damage. Patients may be hemiplegic, dysphasic, and disoriented. Early rehabilitation is critical to help the patient return to a functional existence as soon as possible.

BRAIN DEATH

Definition

The diagnosis of brain death is not difficult to make in terms of testing, but it may be extremely difficult for a practitioner to accept. A declaration of brain death has been necessitated by medicine's ability through technology to keep the heart beating and the respiratory system functioning even though the brain has no ability to recover. Brain death is defined as "irreversible cessation of all functions of the entire brain including the brainstem" (President's Commission for the Study of Ethical Problems in Medicine and Biomedical Behavioral Research, 1981).

Clinical Findings

The diagnosis is generally based on physical findings, including the absence of brainstem reflexes, absence of cortical activity, and the establishment of the irreversibility of the condition. (President's Commission for the Study of Ethical Problems in Medicine and Biomedical Behavioral Research, 1981).

Radiologic Appearance

Pancerebral angiography is helpful in determining the absence of cortical activity and establishing irreversibility of the condition. This test is used primarily in situations in which suppressant drugs such as high dose barbiturates have been administered (Marshall et al, 1990). A lack of intracranial

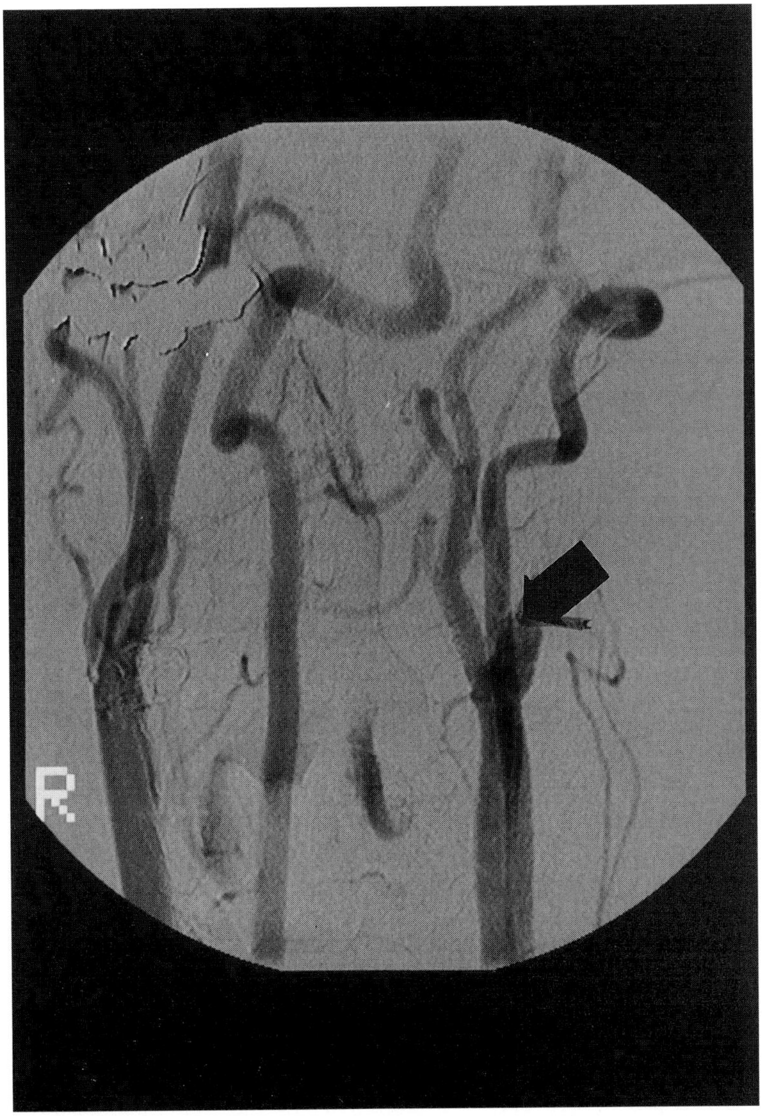

Fig. 4-11 Cerebral vascular accident secondary to a blood clot formation. This arch cerebral angiogram shows an occlusion of the left internal carotid artery. Notice the stump-like appearance of the left internal carotid artery, which does not extend up into the head like the right internal carotid artery.

blood flow from each of the four major vessels supplying the brain is an absolute indication of brain death.

Radionucleotide scanning of the cerebral circulation following injection of an appropriate radionucleotide is also evidence of brain death (Fig. 4-12). The advantages of this cerebral blood flow test are that it can be done at the bedside and that it is less expensive and less cumbersome than pancerebral angiography (Marshall et al, 1990). The only disadvantage of radionucleotide scanning is that it can only adequately measure carotid arterial flow.

Other neurological injuries and problems

SWELLING—DIFFUSE BRAIN INJURY (INCREASED INTRACRANIAL PRESSURE)

Definition

Increased intracranial pressure (ICP) is caused by a variety of neurologic problems such as head trauma, brain tumors, hemorrhage, cerebral edema, increased cerebral spinal fluid volume, and some metabolic dysfunctions. The cause of the swelling and increased ICP must be determined expeditiously so that treatment can be started.

Clinical Findings

The patient will have a loss of consciousness and a score of 8 or less on the Glasgow Coma scale. Depending on how high the pressure rises, the patient may exhibit the following signs of herniation: a fixed dilated pupil, posturing or a flaccid motor response, a rising systolic blood pressure, a widened pulse pressure, and bradycardia.

Radiologic Appearance

X-ray films are of little help in diagnosing increased ICP. As mentioned previously, if the pressure elevation is long standing, the skull may show signs of erosion and thinning. If the pressure increase is related to an epidural hemorrhage, a fracture of the temporal bone may be seen. If the ICP is sufficiently high, the midline structure of the pineal gland may be displaced, especially if a lesion on one side of the brain is causing the rise in pressure. The pineal gland would be pushed to the side opposite of the lesion.

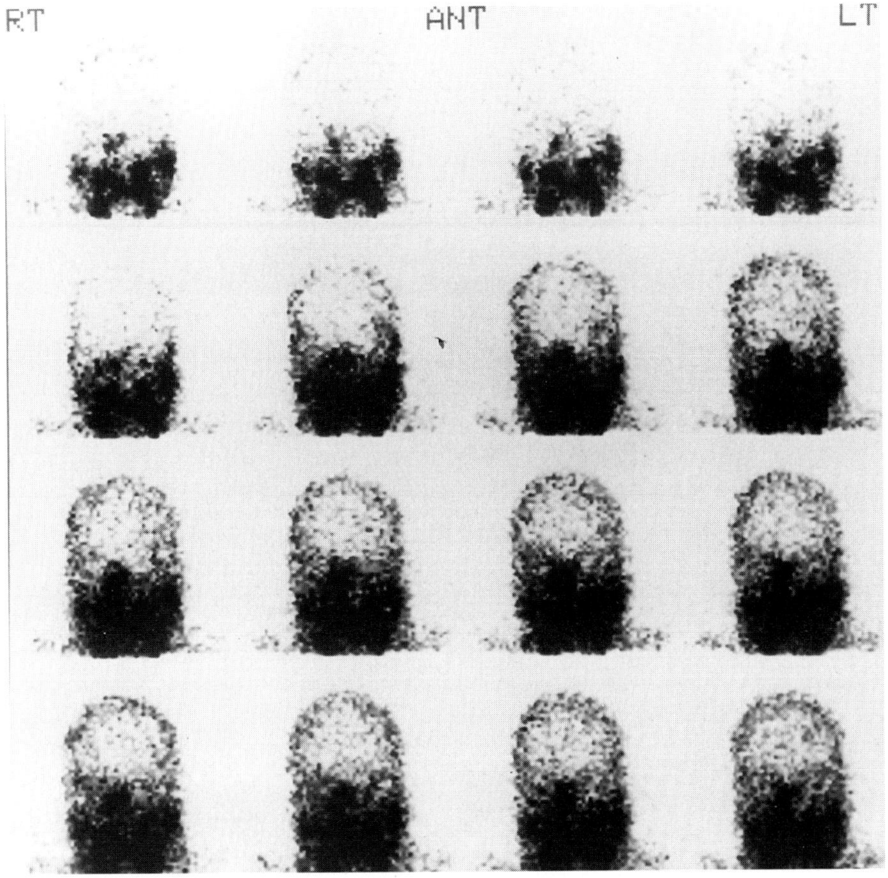

A

Fig. 4-12 **A** and **B,** Brain death. Nuclear blood flow study clinically compatible with brain death. There is no flow of blood to the brain in the center of the head. Notice that there is still blood flow to the scalp.

Continued.

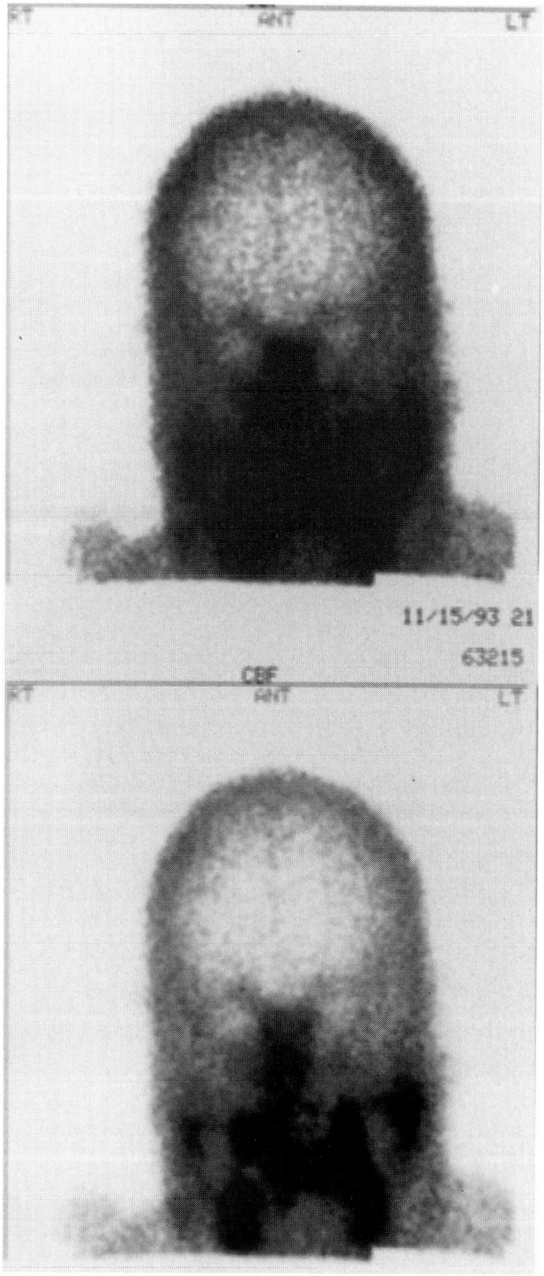

B

Fig. 4-12, cont'd

The CT scan is widely recognized as the most valuable tool for diagnosing increased ICP as well as the potential cause for it. The CT scan reliably shows any shifts caused by brain swelling and impending herniation (Fig. 4-13). The ventricular system can be easily viewed on the CT scan, and the pressure on the ventricles produces smaller than normal ventricles (slit ventricles) (Fig. 4-14). If a ventriculostomy has been done to relieve CSF pressure and/or to monitor the ICP in a patient, the placement of the ventriculostomy catheter can be checked by skull or CT scan (Fig. 4-15). The catheter is radiopaque, so it appears on the film as a white tube placed into the ventricle. In the future, magnetic resonance imaging (MRI) may be used to find the cause of the raised ICP; it can show shearing of white matter and differentiate the type of cerebral edema better than the CT scan (Marshall et al, 1990).

Nursing Implications

The head of the patient's bed is usually elevated to 30 degrees at all times for patients with increased ICP. During a CT scan the patient will be flat for a long period of time, which may raise the ICP during and following the scan. The management of the patient with increased ICP is complex. The traditional therapies to prevent or control ICP include mechanical ventilation with hyperventilation to maintain the arterial carbon dioxide tension ($PaCO_2$) between 27 and 33 mm Hg, osmotic diuretic therapy with mannitol and/or systemic diuretics such as furosemide, and control of the patient's cerebral metabolic rate with barbiturates or sedation. Much nursing research has focused on the effects of nursing care on ICP. Results of this research have brought some changes in nursing care. These changes include hyperoxygenation and hyperventilation before and after suctioning, elevation of the head of the bed, and awareness of the cumulative effects of nursing care on ICP. Close neurologic assessment and monitoring is critical to detect changes in the ICP and neurologic function. If the patient has a ventriculostomy for monitoring and drainage, the nurse should inspect the insertion site for the signs and symptoms of infection and sample the CSF frequently for cultures.

SKULL FRACTURES

Definition

Skull fractures are one of the most common forms of head injury. They are classified according to type: linear, comminuted, depressed, and basal skull.

A

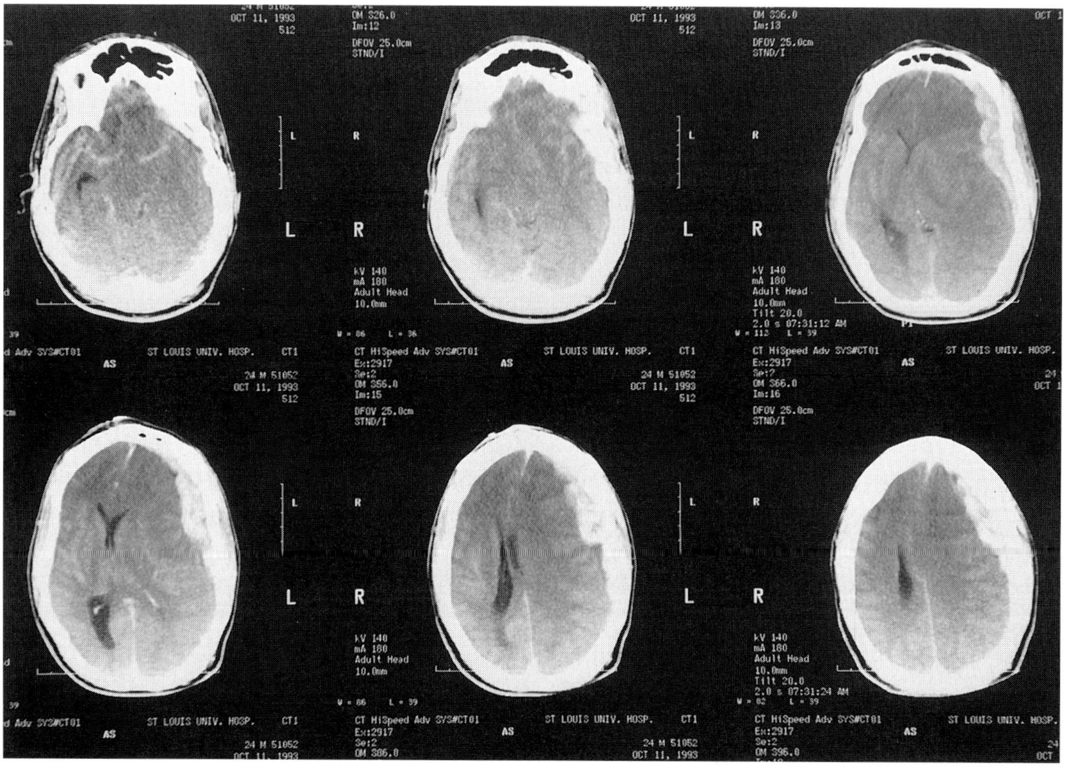

Fig. 4-13 **A** and **B,** Increased ICP—midline shift. This patient has a left-to-right shift of brain tissue, secondary to an acute subdural hematoma with subfascial herniation. In the top left window of the CT notice the presence of subarachnoid blood along the falx cerebelli and the compressed ventricles (a clearer view is in close-up in Fig. 4-14).

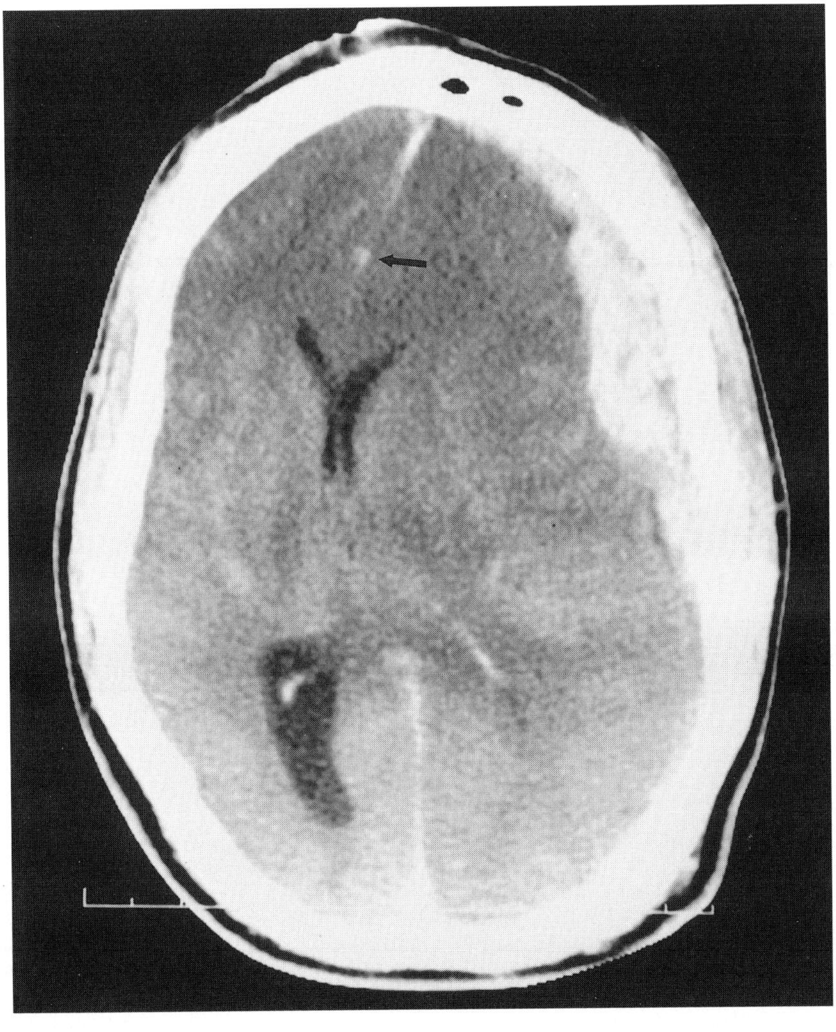
B

Fig. 4-13, cont'd

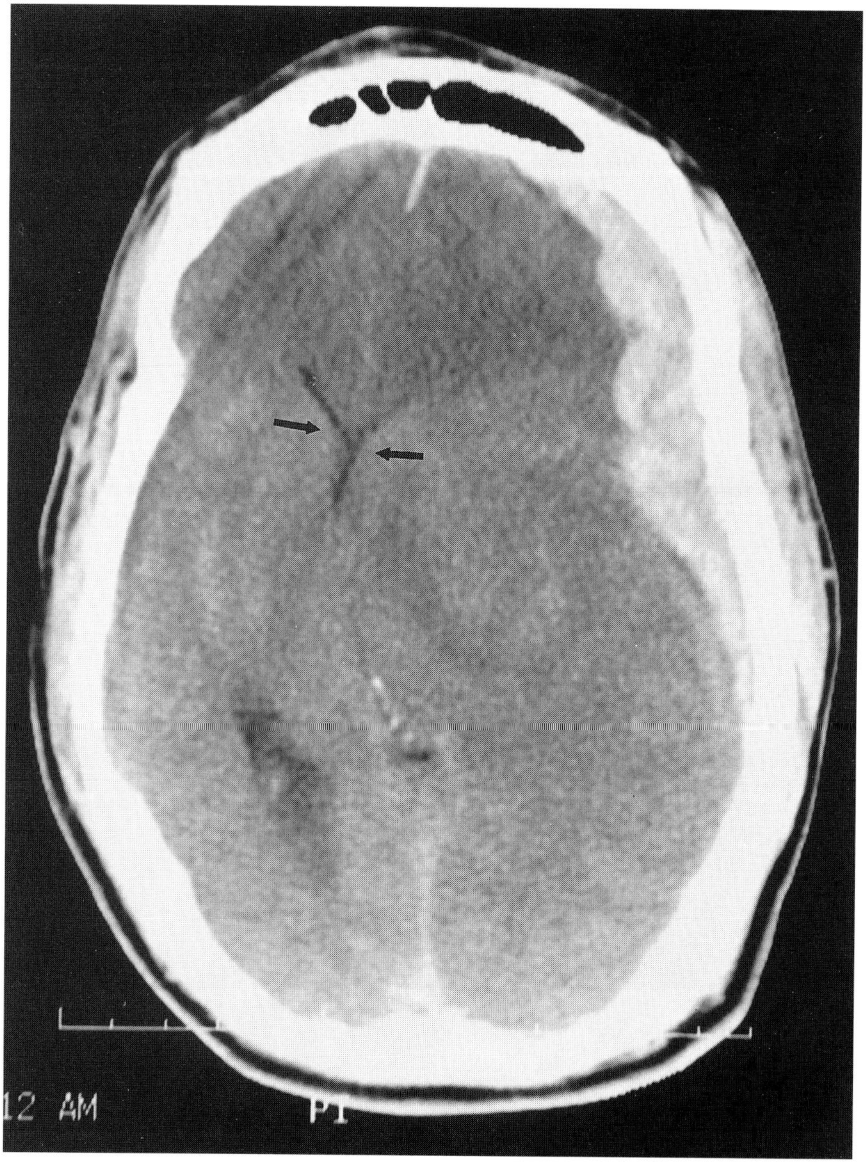

Fig. 4-14 Increased ICP—compressed ventricles. Slit-like ventricular horns are a sign of increased intracranial pressure. Noticc the midline shift. This is the same patient as pictured in Fig. 4-13.

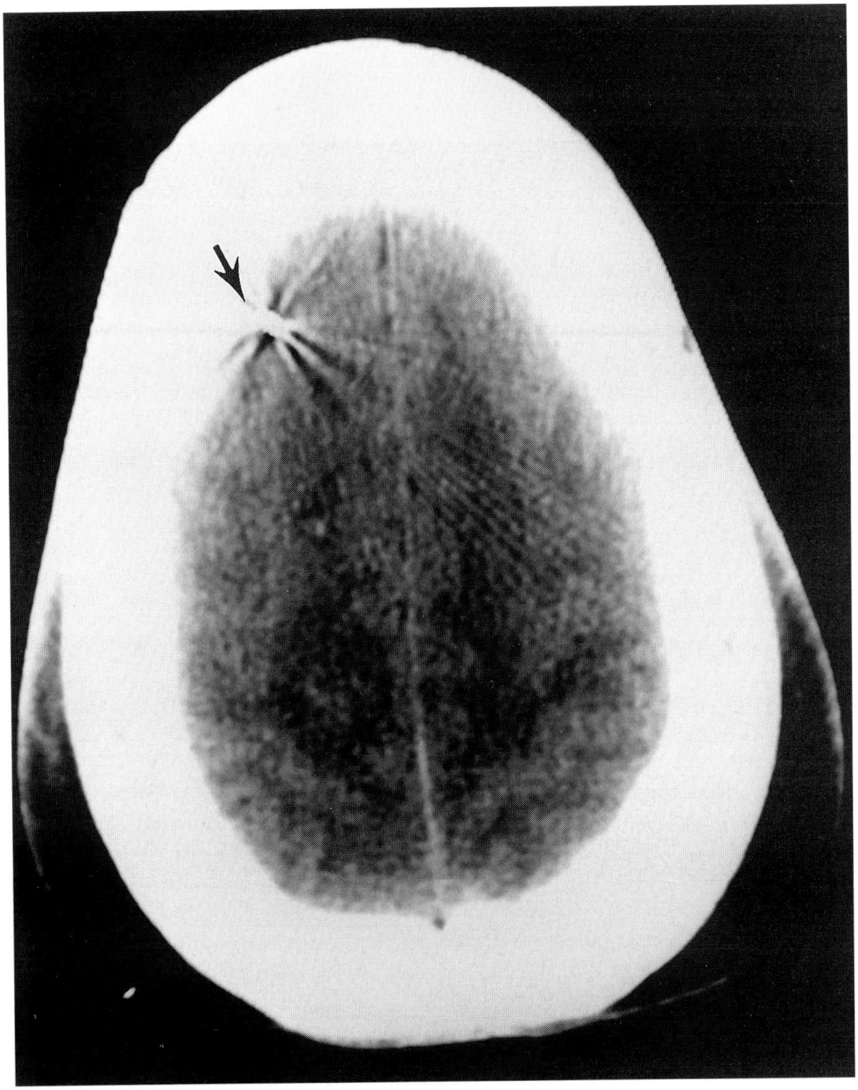
A

Fig. 4-15 Ventriculostomy/fiberoptic catheters for increased ICP. **A,** ICP monitor situated at the right frontal area. Notice how the metal causes artifact.

Continued.

B

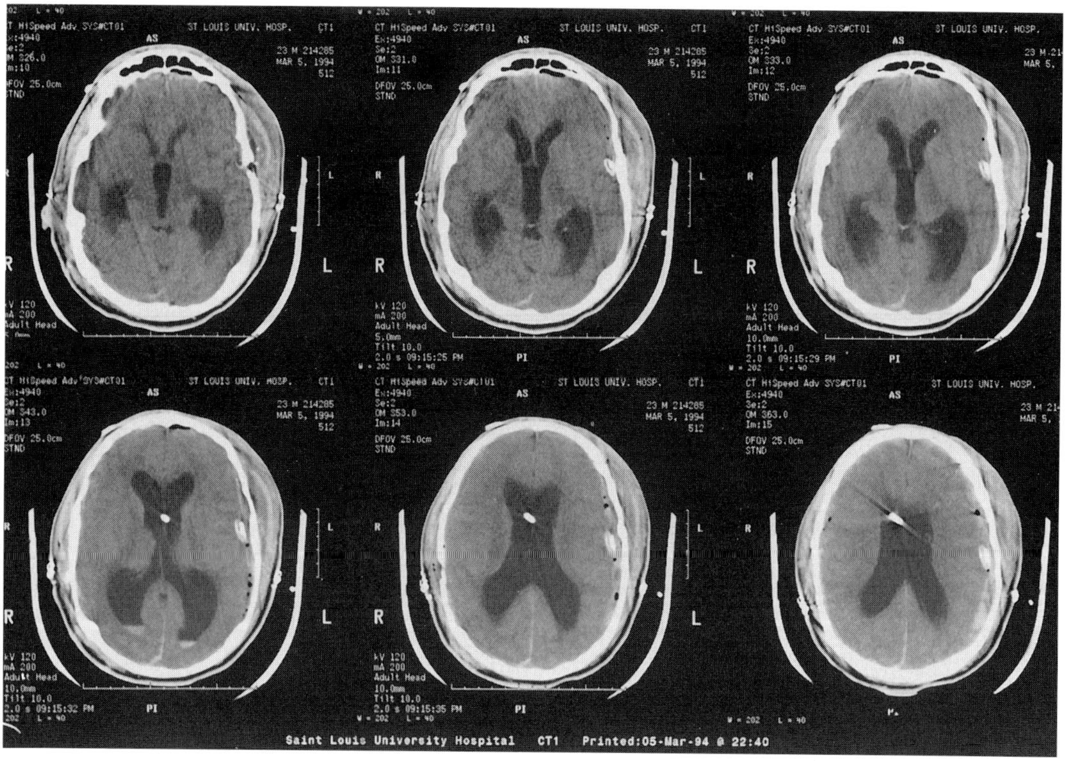

Fig. 4-15, cont'd. Ventriculostomy/fiberoptic catheters for increased ICP. **B** and **C,** This is a typical example of hydrocephalus with an intraventricular catheter (i.e., ventriculostomy) in place in the frontal horns of the lateral ventricle, which appears as a bright white spot. Also notice the small pneumocephali (dark circles) on the left side, a common postoperative finding.

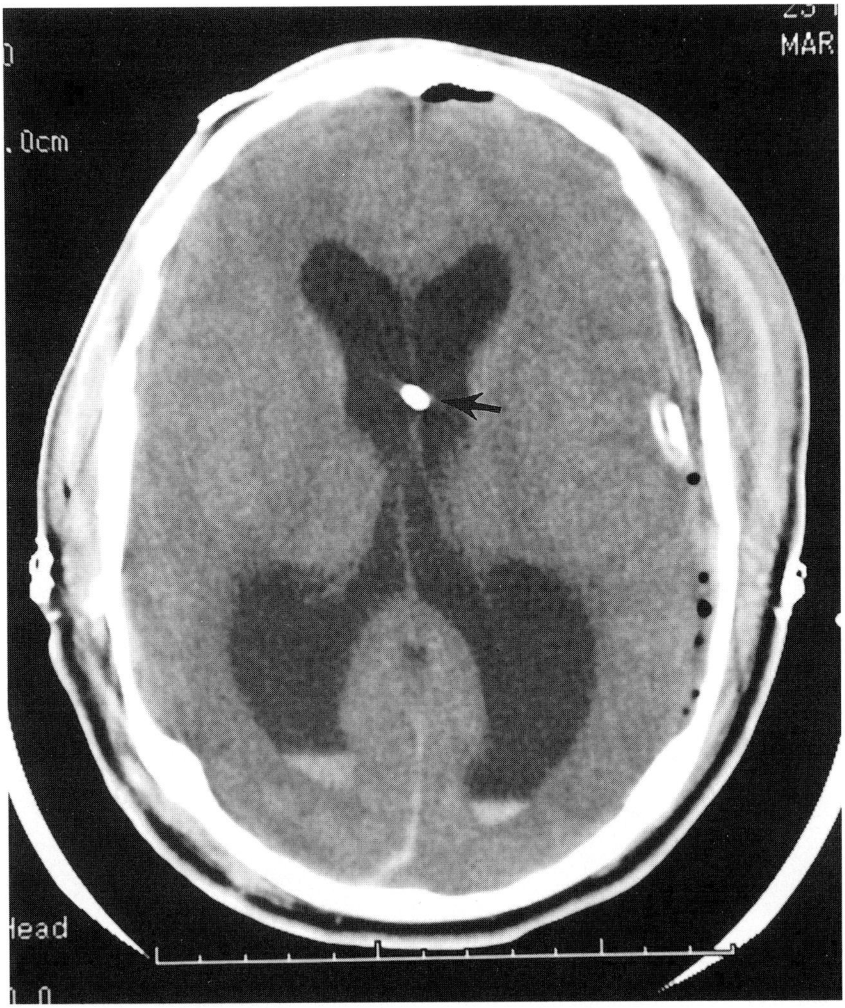

C

Fig. 4-15, cont'd. C, For legend see opposite page.

Continued.

D

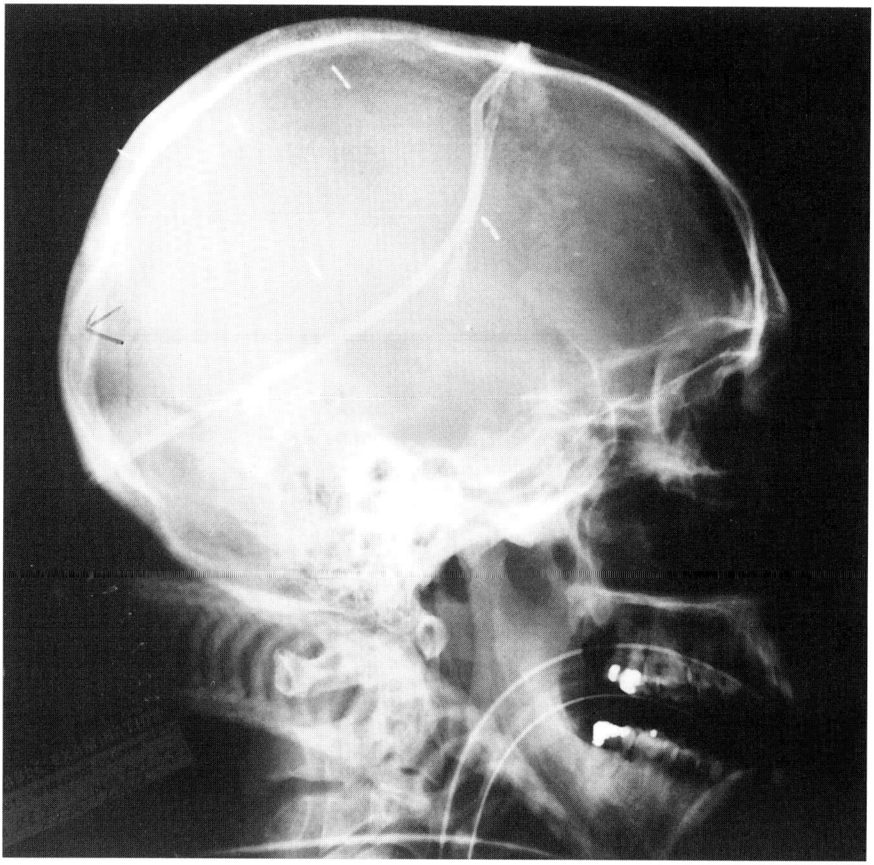

Fig. 4-15, cont'd. Ventriculostomy/fiberoptic catheters for increased ICP. **D,** A plain film showing a ventricular catheter in place. Also notice the occipital fracture and endotracheal tube.

The type of fracture that occurs depends on the velocity, direction, and momentum of the object that causes the injury.

Clinical Findings

The signs and symptoms of skull fractures vary with the type of fracture. Most patients with linear fractures have no neurologic findings unless the middle meningeal artery is disrupted by the fracture. Depending on the depth of the depressed fracture, the patient may have no neurologic deficit or the patient may be comatose. Seizures are also frequently observed in patients with depressed fractures that are deep enough to injure the underlying tissue.

The patient with a basal skull fracture may have drainage of CSF from the nose (rhinorrhea) or ear (otorrhea). In addition to rhinorrhea, the patient with a frontal bone fracture will also have "raccoon's eyes" (bilateral ecchymosis of the eyes). Battle's sign (bruising of the mastoid bone) indicates an injury to the mastoid portion of the temporal bone. Neurologically these patients are usually awake.

Radiologic Appearance

Linear fractures appear on the radiograph as cracks in the skull and account for about 75% of all skull fractures. Temporal bone fractures may be associated with epidural hematomas. A comminuted fracture is a shattering or fragmentation of the skull. Multiple fracture lines are seen on skull radiographs. With a depressed skull fracture the skull pushes inward toward the brain and may actually compress brain tissue. A depressed skull fracture is also easily visible on a CT scan (Fig. 4-16). A basilar skull fracture occurs at the base of the skull. The fracture usually arises from an extension of a linear fracture, especially frontal and temporal bones, and involves paranasal sinuses or mastoid sinuses, which appear black on the film (air is seen in the sinuses) (Marshall et al, 1990) (Fig. 4-17).

Nursing Implications

A depressed skull fracture is considered a "dirty" injury because hair, dirt, and pieces of impacting objects may be found in the wound. Surgical elevation of the bone is usually required. With a basilar skull fracture, the fractures through the sinuses leak through the nose (rhinorrhea), the ear (otorrhea), or postnasally, causing infections such as meningitis.

A

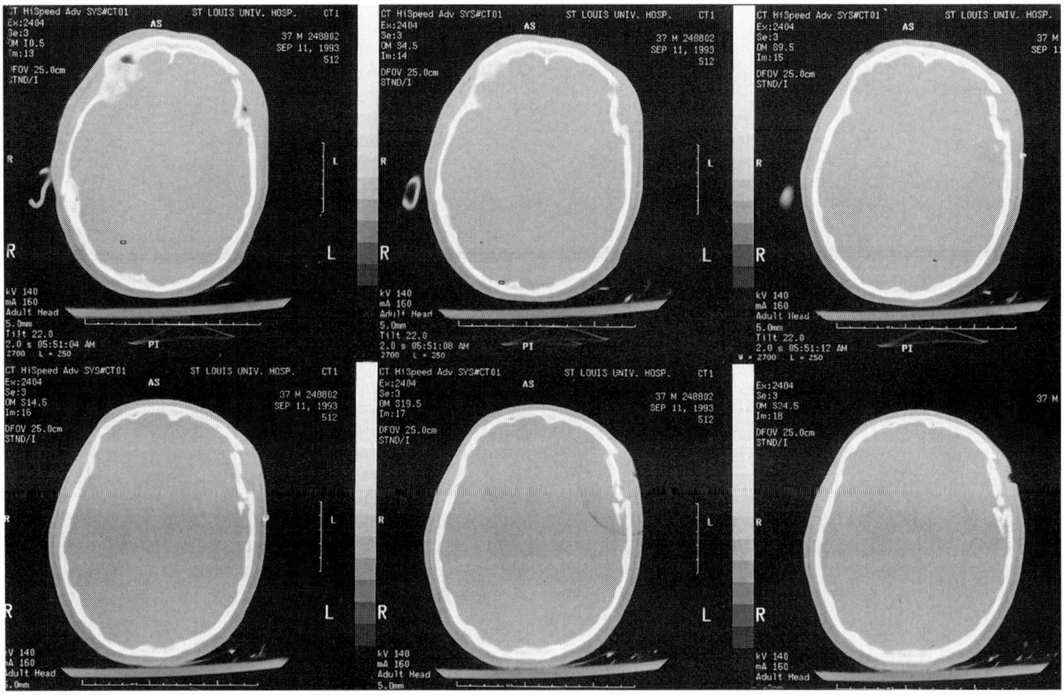

Fig. 4-16 **A** and **B,** Depressed skull fracture. A bone window of an axial CT scan showing a depressed skull fracture of the left frontal area. Notice the bone fragments.

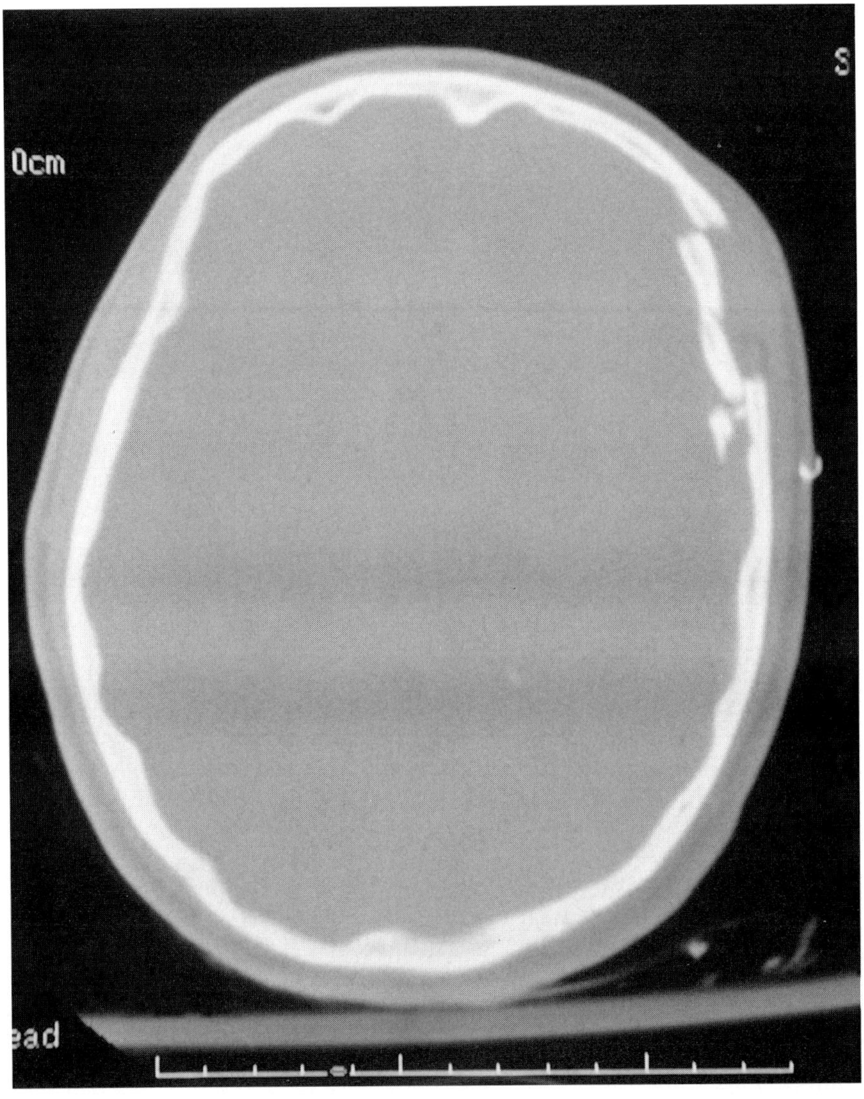

B

Fig. 4-16, cont'd

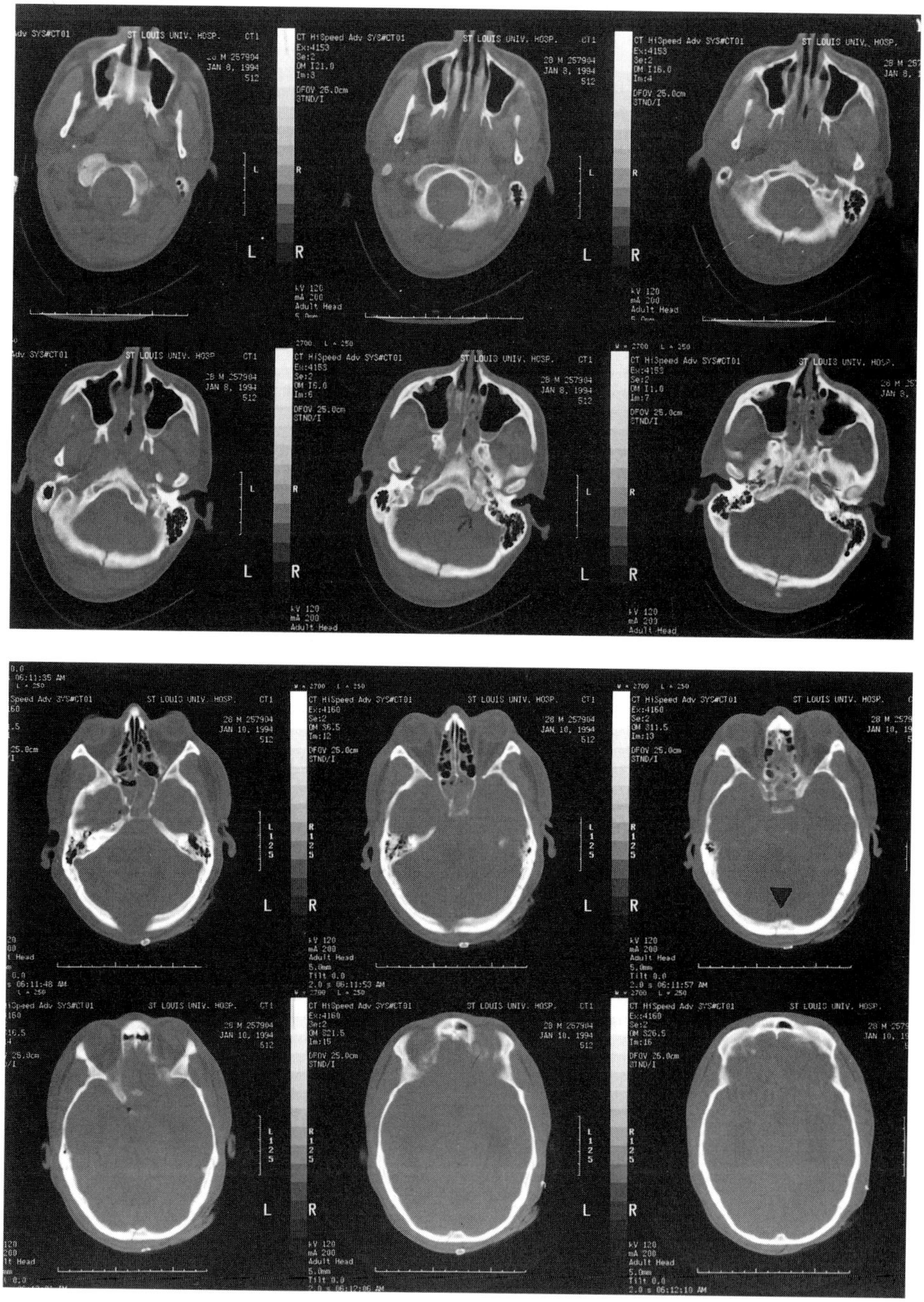

A

B

Fig. 4-17 **A** through **D,** Basilar skull fracture. These views of a CT scan show fractures at the base of the skull and the foramen magnum.

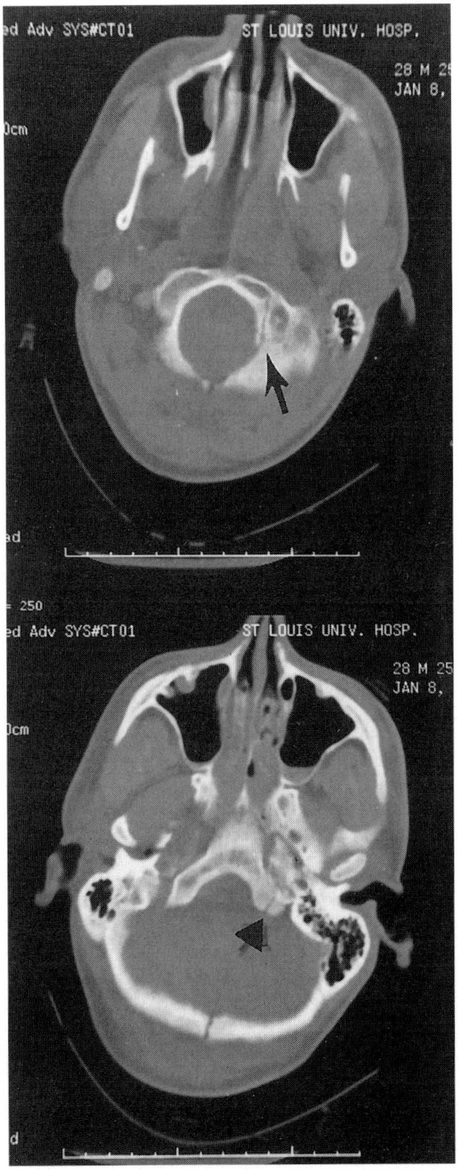

C

Fig. 4-17, cont'd

Continued.

D

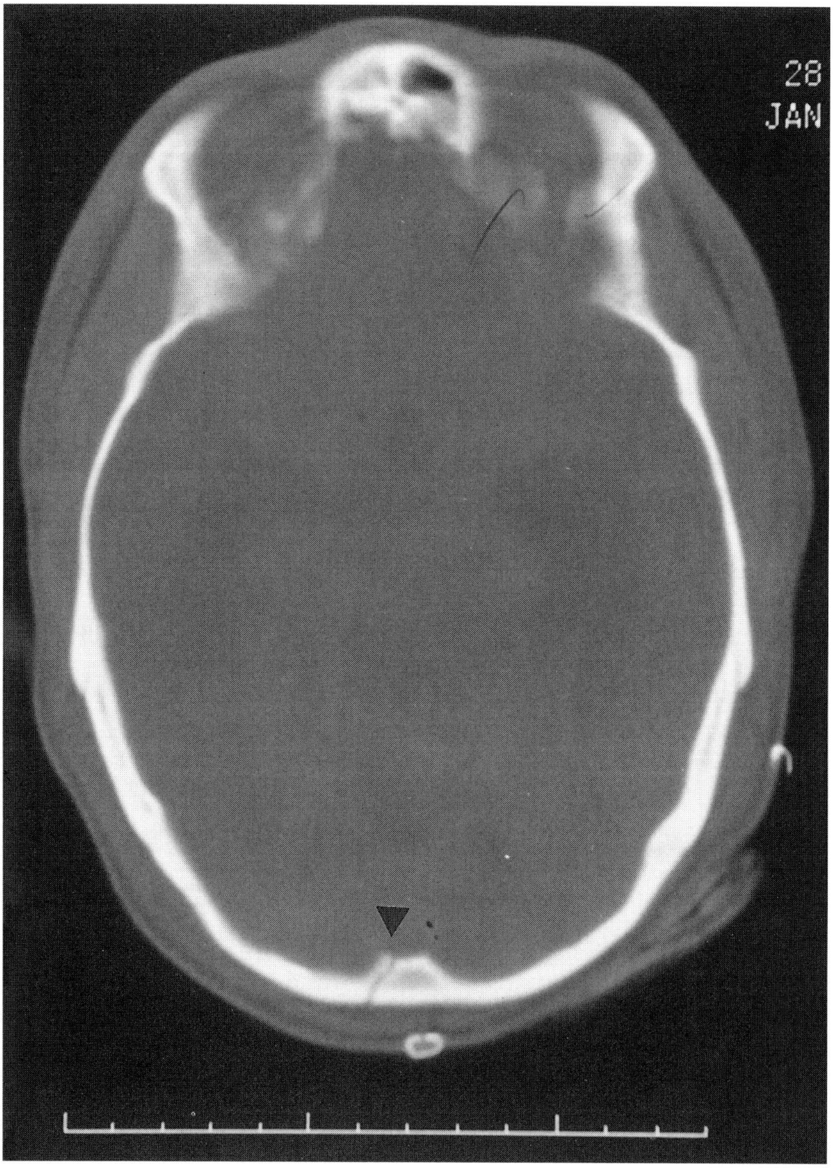

Fig. 4-17, cont'd

FACIAL INJURIES

Definition

Injuries to the face can be the result of motor vehicle accidents, falls, assaults, or sporting events. The incidence of these injuries is high. The box on p. 167 lists the major bones of the face divided into thirds. Midface fractures are the most common because of the immobility of this part of the face.

Clinical Findings

The face will usually appear distorted following an injury. Considerable bleeding is associated with facial injuries because of the rich blood supply in that area. If the mandible and maxilla are affected, the patient's airway may be compromised. Pain is usually associated with facial injuries.

Radiologic Appearance

Fractures are easily identified on a radiograph. Midface fractures are classified by the extent of facial bone involvement. The original classification was done in 1901 by LeFort. A LeFort I fracture involves a horizontal line that separates the maxillary alveolus from the upper part of the face. A LeFort II fracture is a pyramid-shaped separation involving the nasomaxillary segment of the zygomatic and orbital portions of the midface. The separation of the facial bones from the cranium through the orbits and naso-ethmoid areas is a LeFort III fracture (Tessler, 1977) (Fig. 4-18).

The nasal bones sustain a high number of injuries because of their prominence. Nasal fractures can be classified into three major categories: depressed, laterally angulated, and comminuted (Deli and Bower, 1988).

Mandibular fractures usually occur because of blunt trauma to the face. The mandible's shape allows it to fracture easily in two places. The body of the mandible and the condylar-subcondylar areas are frequently displaced. The AP and lateral oblique x-ray films of the mandible are used in the diagnosis of a fracture.

Nursing Implications

Managing the patient's bleeding when positioning the patient for the radiographs is important. Close attention should be paid to the patient's ability to manage secretions while lying flat.

A

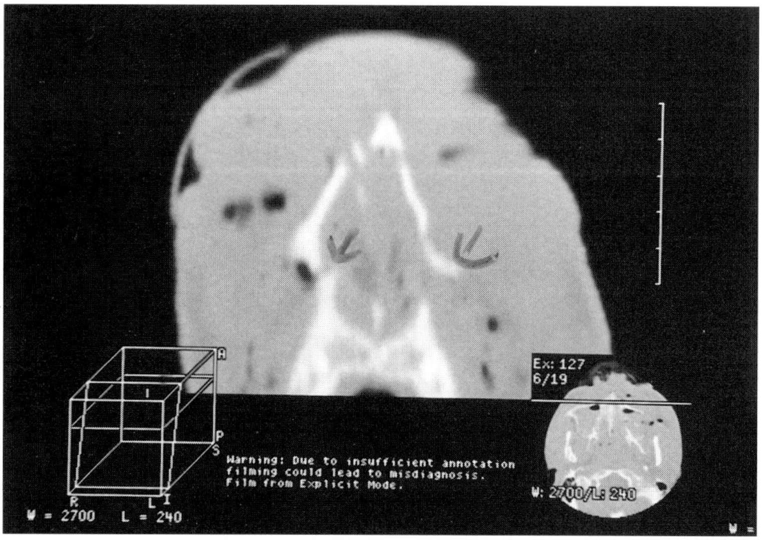

B

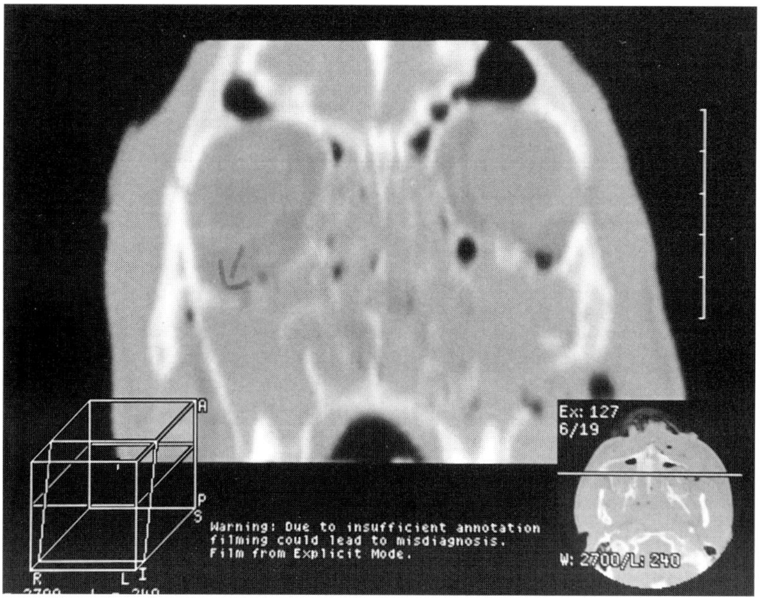

Fig. 4-18 **A** and **B,** LeFort fracture. A cut coronal view through the nasal septum shows bilateral nasal fractures. There is also a fracture of the orbital floor on the right side and the lateral wall. These findings are consistent with a LeFort fracture.

BONES OF THE FACE

UPPER THIRD	MIDDLE THIRD	LOWER THIRD
Frontal bone	Superior orbital fissure	Body of mandible
Glabella	Inferior orbital fissure	Base of mandible
Supraorbital margin	Zygomatic bone	Alveolar with teeth
Supraorbital notch	Zygomatic process	Mental protuberance
Temporal bone	Body of maxilla	
Nasal bone	Alveolar process with teeth	
Lacrimal bone	Nasal septum-vomer	
Ethmoid bone		

Almost all facial fractures require some form of surgery to correct the deformities. External fixation devices are also helpful in allowing proper healing to occur. A patient with a LeFort II or a LeFort III fracture may also experience a CSF rhinorrhea; nasal packs should be avoided.

ORBITAL FRACTURE

Definition

Fracture of the zygoma always involves the orbit of the eye. LeFort II and LeFort III fractures also involve fractures through the orbits. Blow-out fractures are the result of a spike in intraorbital pressure causing a fracture at the orbital floor or medial wall.

Clinical Findings

The patient will generally have an obvious deformity of the orbit. Pain, edema, and ecchymosis of or bilateral to the affected orbit are also present. The patient may complain of diplopia, and ophthalmoplegia may be found on assessment. In addition to the above symptoms, a sinking of the globe and conjunctival hemorrhage occurs with a blow-out fracture. Blindness caused by a detached retina may occur.

Radiologic Appearance

Radiographs of the face will show fractures of the orbit. Tomography of the orbit will be performed to look at the extent of the orbit disruption. A CT scan will show the fracture as well as the amount of soft tissue injury (Fig. 4-19).

Nursing Implications

The considerations for the patient with an orbital fracture are the same as those for the patient with any facial injury. Protecting the globe is important during tomographic radiographs. Assessment of the patient's ability to see and move the eyes in all spheres is imperative before and following diagnostic studies. Pain may be severe, and the patient may require narcotic analgesia. With a blow-out fracture, the globe should be protected from further injury.

SINUSITIS

Definition

Infection of the sinuses may be caused by an open, traumatic injury, such as with an open skull fracture. Sinusitis is also seen frequently in patients who have been nasally intubated. Sinusitis can lead to subdural empyema (subdural abscess).

Clinical Findings

The nurse may observe drainage from the patient's nose or ears. The patient may have a history of chronic sinusitis. The patient experiences localized pain over the sinuses (the brow and between the eyes or over the mastoid processes). Tenderness and swelling of these areas are also present. If the infection spreads to the subdural space, the patient may experience severe headache, fever, and vomiting. Focal neurologic deficits can also appear.

Radiologic Appearance

On the radiograph, the affected sinuses are opaque (Fig. 4-20). The extent of the infection can bc observed on a CT scan, especially if subdural space involvement is suspected.

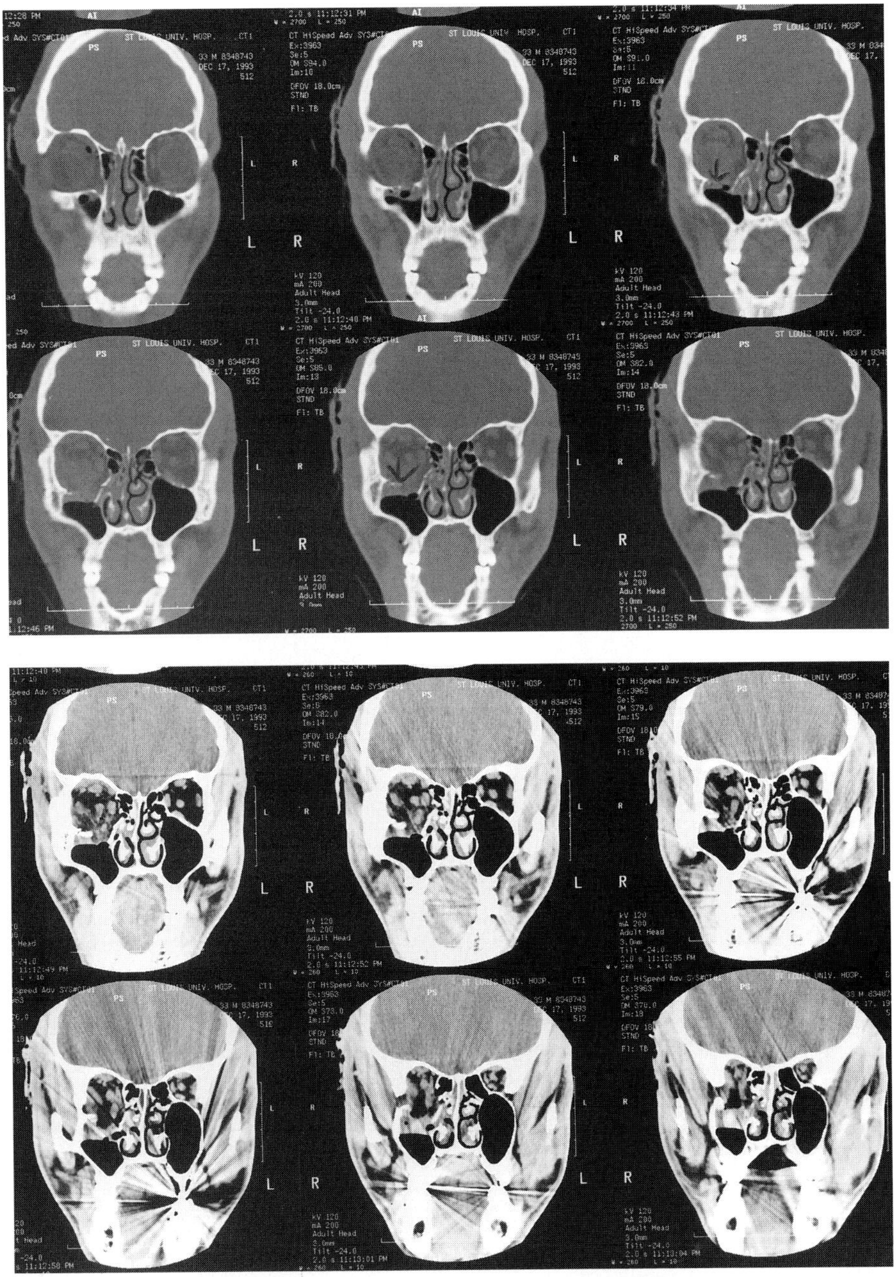

A

B

Fig. 4-19 **A** through **D,** Orbit fracture. CT scan shows a facial fracture involving the inferomedial and floor of the right orbit (see *arrows*). Notice that the right maxillary sinus is less aerated than the left and is partially filled with fluid.

Continued.

C

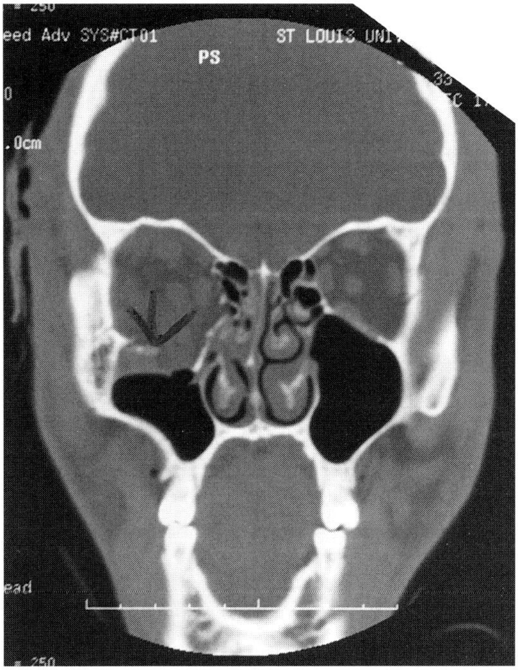

D

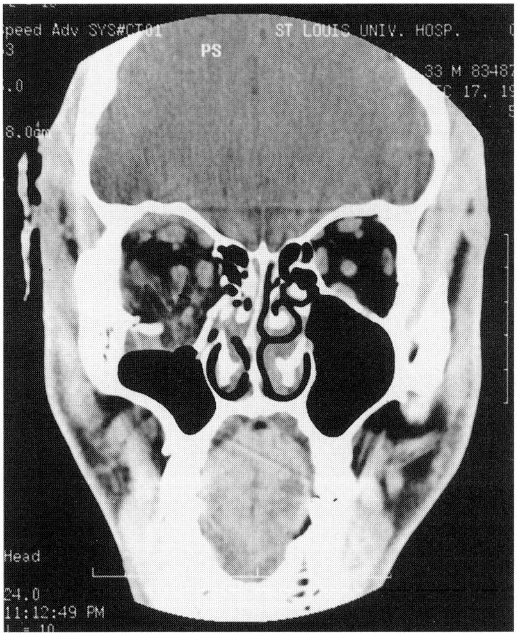

Fig. 4-19, cont'd

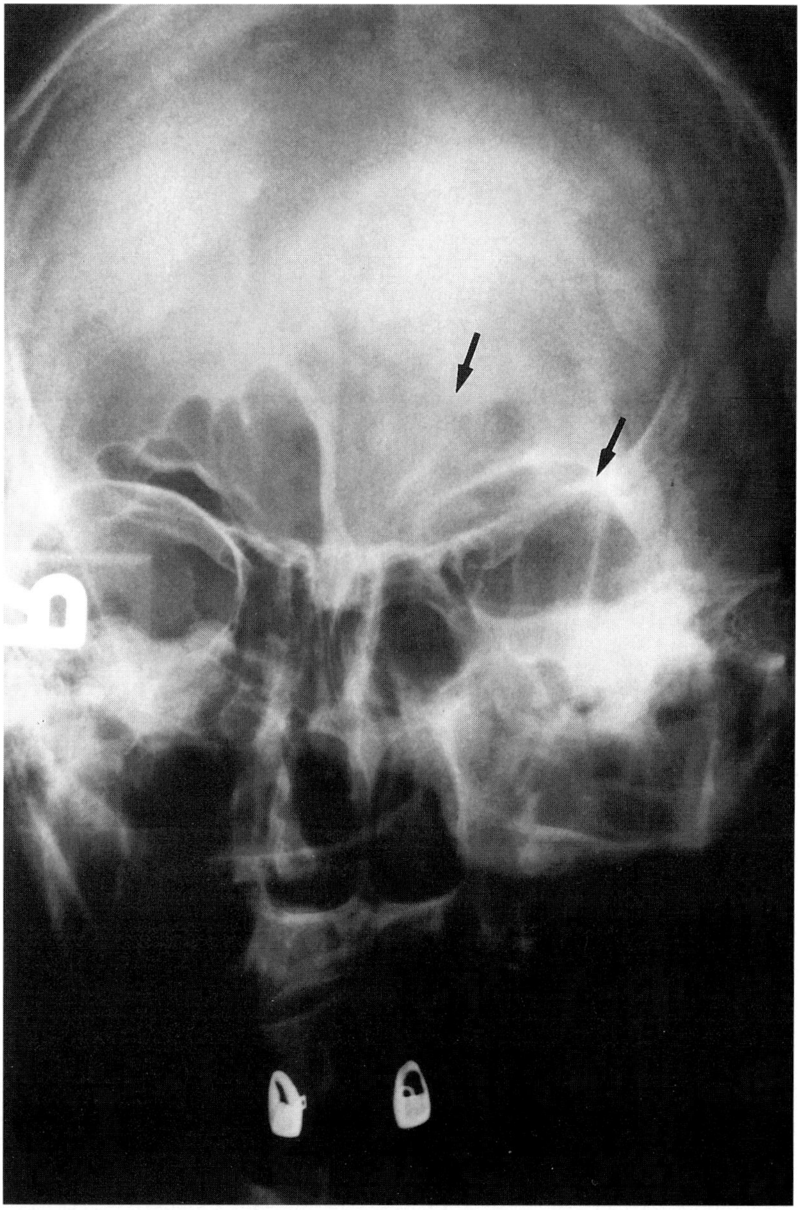

A

Fig. 4-20 **A** and **B,** Sinusitis. Radiographs of the paranasal sinuses reveal opacification of the left maxillary and left frontal sinus. The superior portion of the left frontal sinus has lost its scalloped border and sclerotic rim, possibly suggesting frontal bone osteomyelitis. Notice an excellent view of the odontoid at the triangle in **B.**

Continued.

B

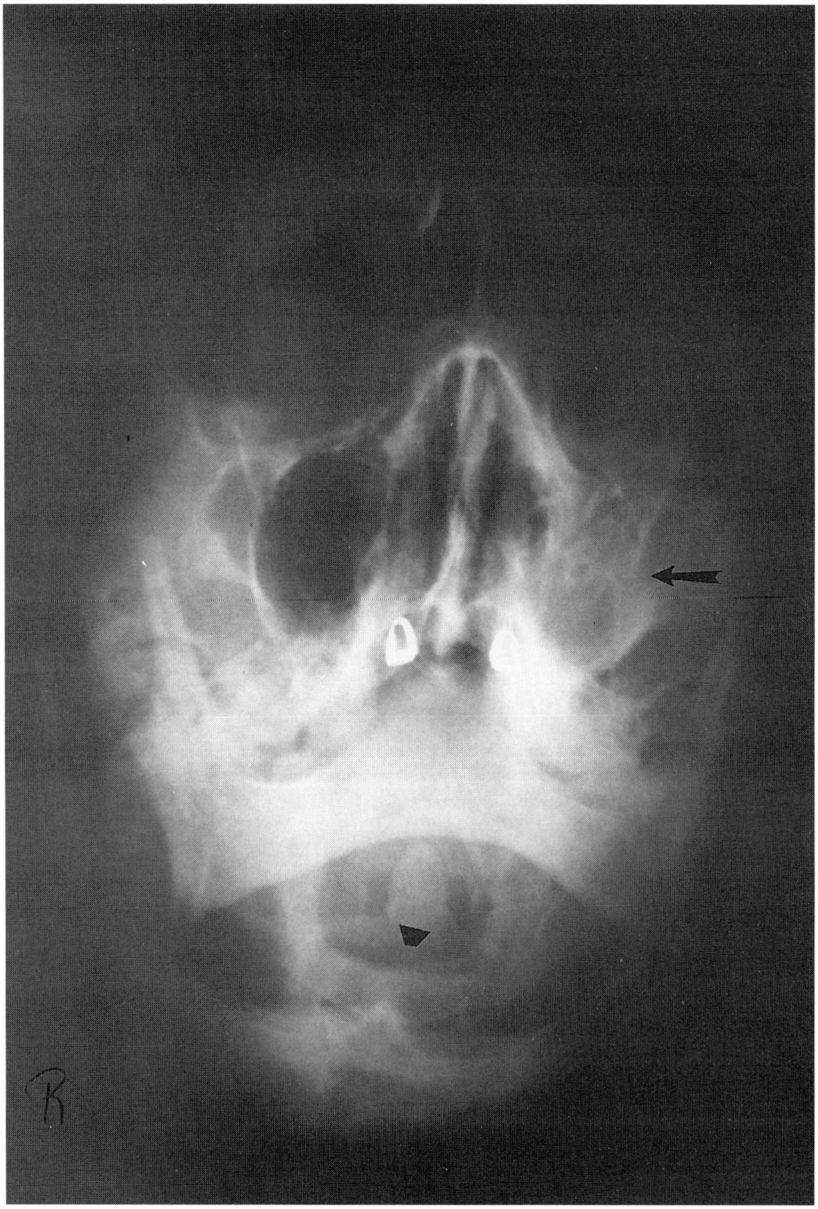

Fig. 4-20, cont'd

Nursing Implications

The nurse should observe the patient for any signs of infection, such as fever, malaise, vomiting, or any signs of pus draining from the nose or ears. A sudden onset of headache may indicate a spread of the infection.

SPINAL INJURIES

Definition

Spinal injuries occur at the rate of 10,000 to 12,000 per year in the United States. In a spinal injury the neurologic damage is usually the result of the movement of the vertebral column. Spinal injuries are generally classified as vertical compression, hyperflexion, flexion-compression, flexion-rotation, hyperextension, and extension-rotation injuries. Compression injuries result in either a wedge compression of the body of the vertebrae or a burst fracture, depending on the forces applied. Injuries are also classified as stable or unstable. With a stable injury, all of the supporting structures, such as ligaments and muscles, are intact, which decreases the risk for further injury. With an unstable injury, the ligaments are disrupted as well as the bony injury.

When viewing the plain radiograph of a compression fracture, the nurse should note a flattening of the vertebral body (Fig. 4-21). The injured body(ies) would be narrow in comparison to the normal body. This injury is best recognized on a lateral film, but can also be seen on an AP film. The body may be intact or show a break with the portions being displaced. Obviously with a fractured body, the potential for further spinal cord damage exists by penetration by the bone fragment.

A spinal cord transection cannot clearly be seen on a radiograph (Fig. 4-22). The term *transection* refers to a physiologic, not physical, transection of the cord. The radiograph would demonstrate a major fracture dislocation of the vertebrae. There may be several millimeters of forward movement of the entire vertebral column, which would compress the entire spinal cord as it tries to continue in a straight line. This fracture often resembles a stair step in appearance with loss of all the supporting ligaments that normally maintain the vertebral column in a straight line.

The subluxation of the vertebrae occurs in a hyperflexion/hypertension type of injury (Fig. 4-23). There is a slight movement of the vertebrae on one another with the ligamentous support remaining intact but stretched. On the

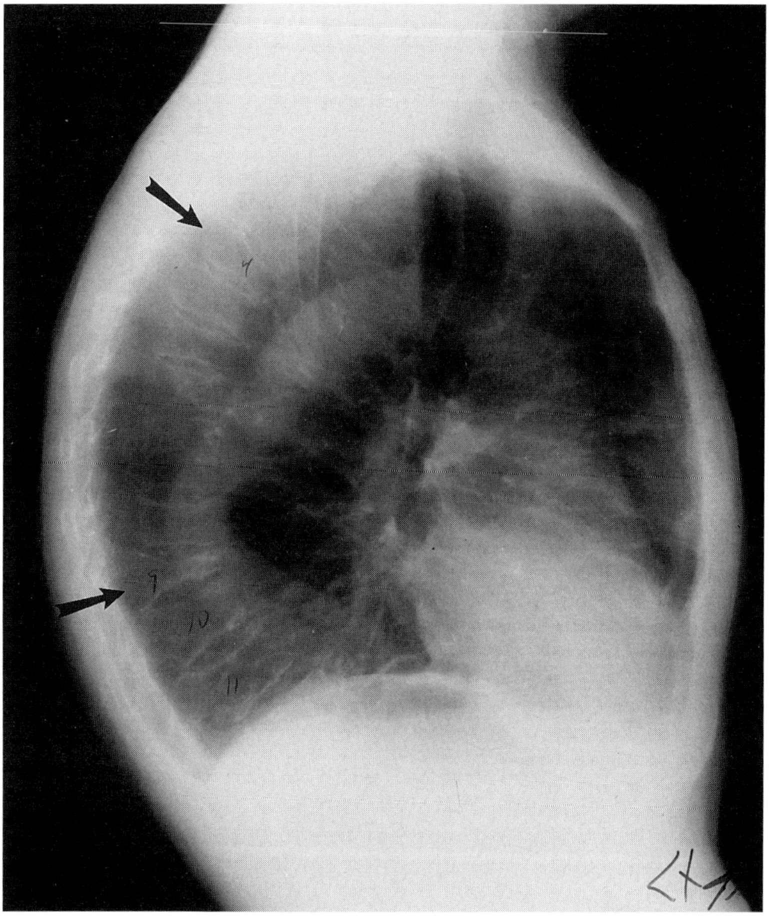

Fig. 4-21 Compression fracture of the spine. This patient has multiple compression fractures from chronic steroid therapy. The *arrows* at T4 and T9 show the vertebrae most affected.

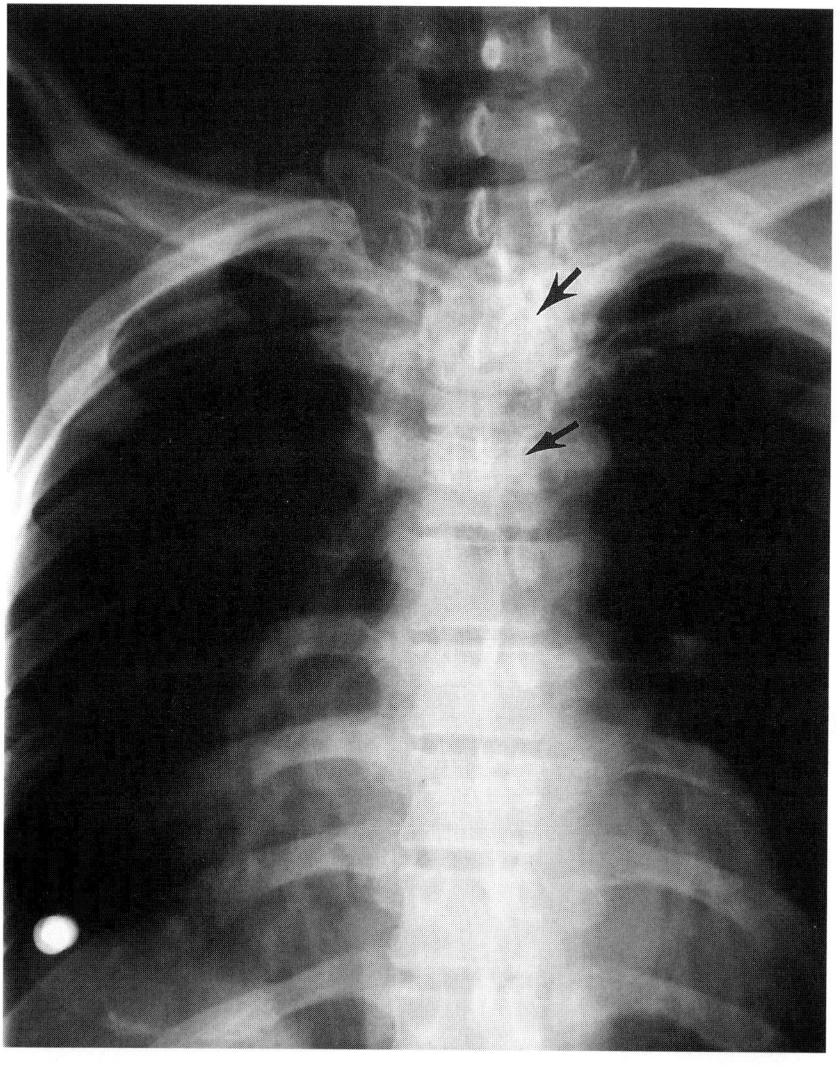

A

Fig. 4-22 **A** through **C,** Spinal fracture/transection. This radiograph demonstrates multiple thoracic vertebral fractures involving T2-4 and proximal ribs T2-5. The CT scan was performed to identify the injury. There was anterior subluxation of T2 on T3. Because of clinical signs an MRI was obtained, which clearly shows complete transection of the spinal cord secondary to a bony fragment occupying the spinal canal at the T2-3 level. Additionally, the MRI demonstrates approximately 50% subluxation of T3 on T4.

Continued.

B

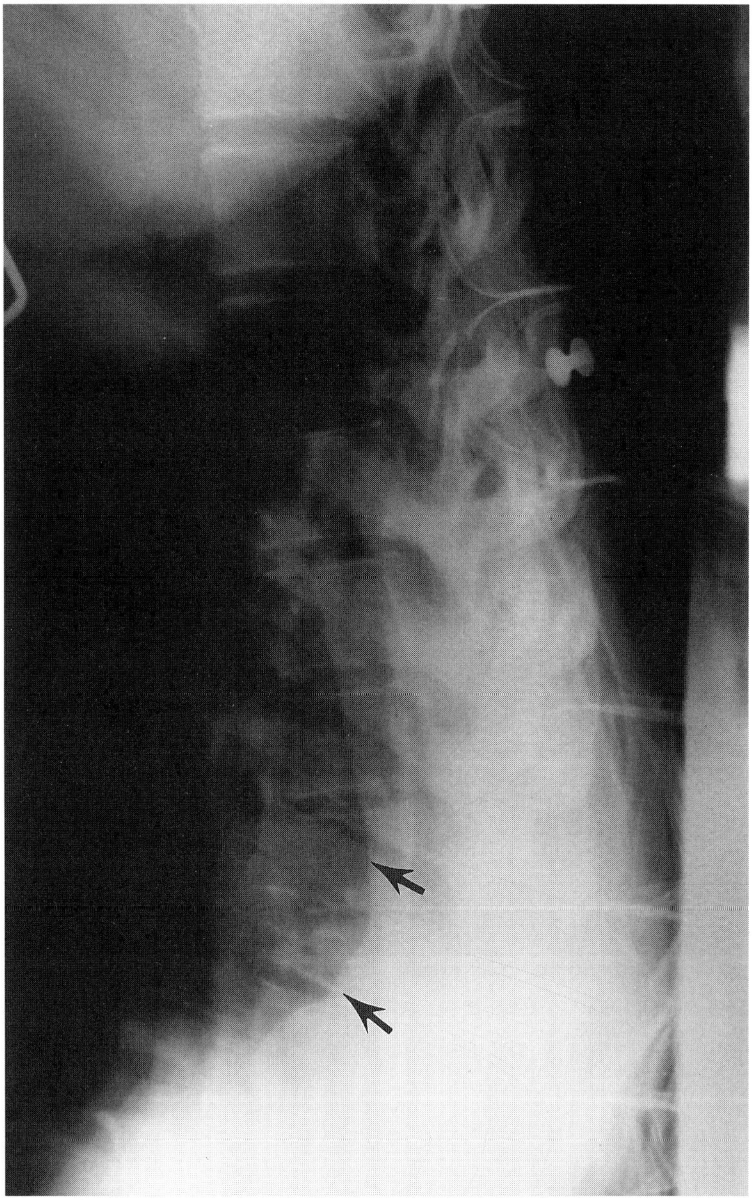

Fig. 4-22, cont'd

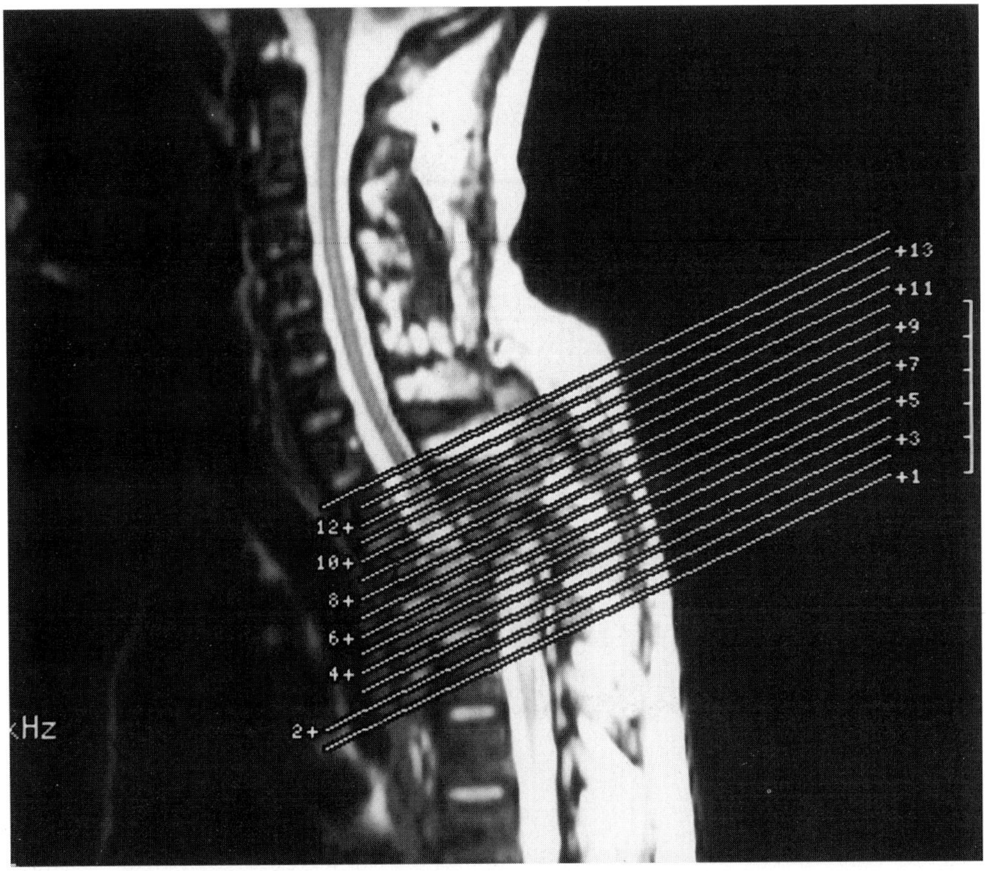

C

Fig. 4-22, cont'd

A

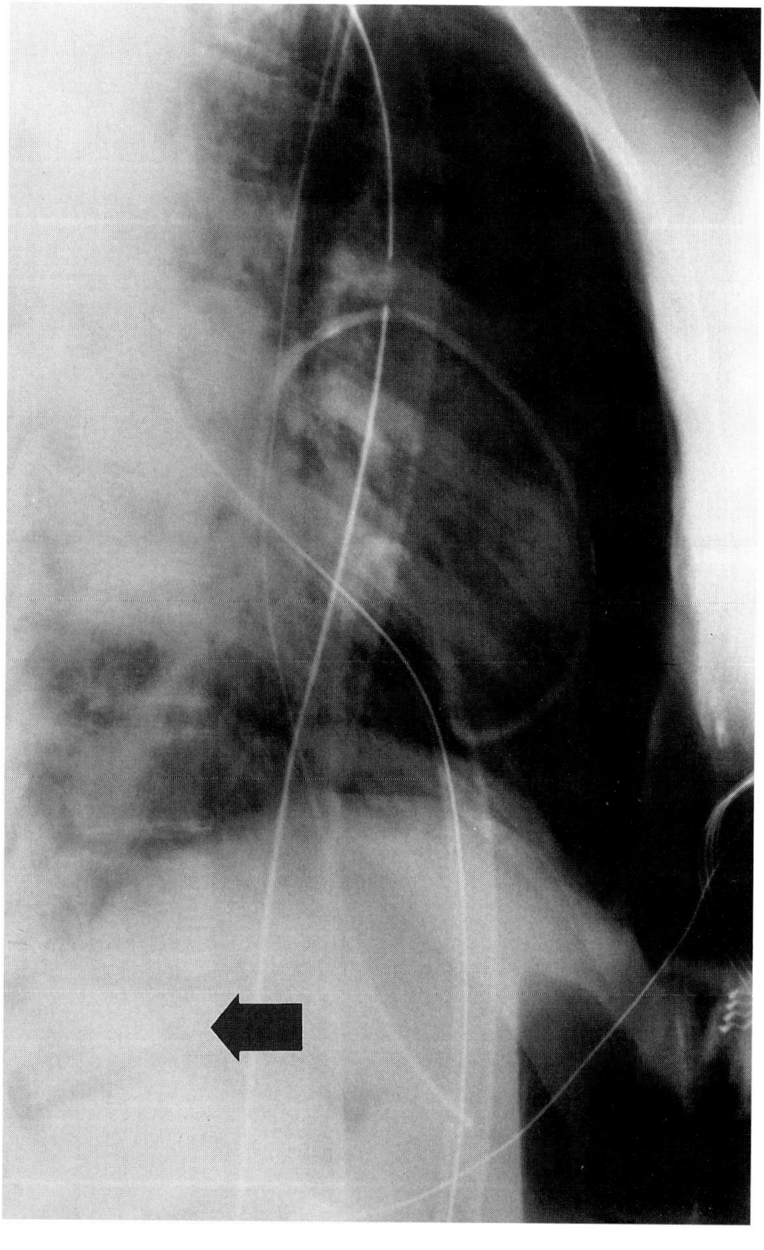

Fig. 4-23 **A** through **C**, Spinal fracture—subluxation. This patient was the victim of an automobile accident. Upright and lateral radiographs of the thoracic and lumbar spine demonstrate approximately a 5 mm subluxation fracture of the lower thoracic vertebrae at approximately the level of T10-12. Also notice the femoral pulmonary artery catheter, bilateral chest tubes, and right lower lung field pulmonary contusion.

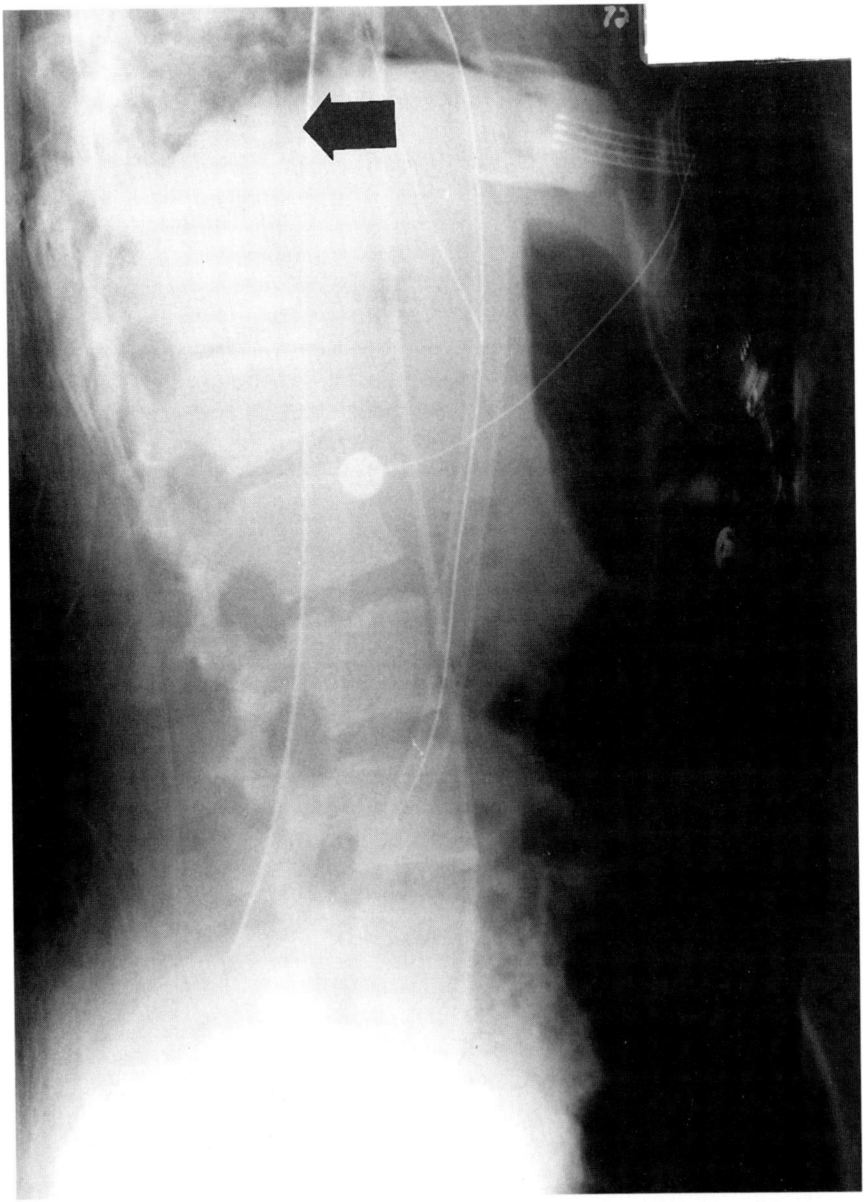

B

Fig. 4-23, cont'd

Continued.

C

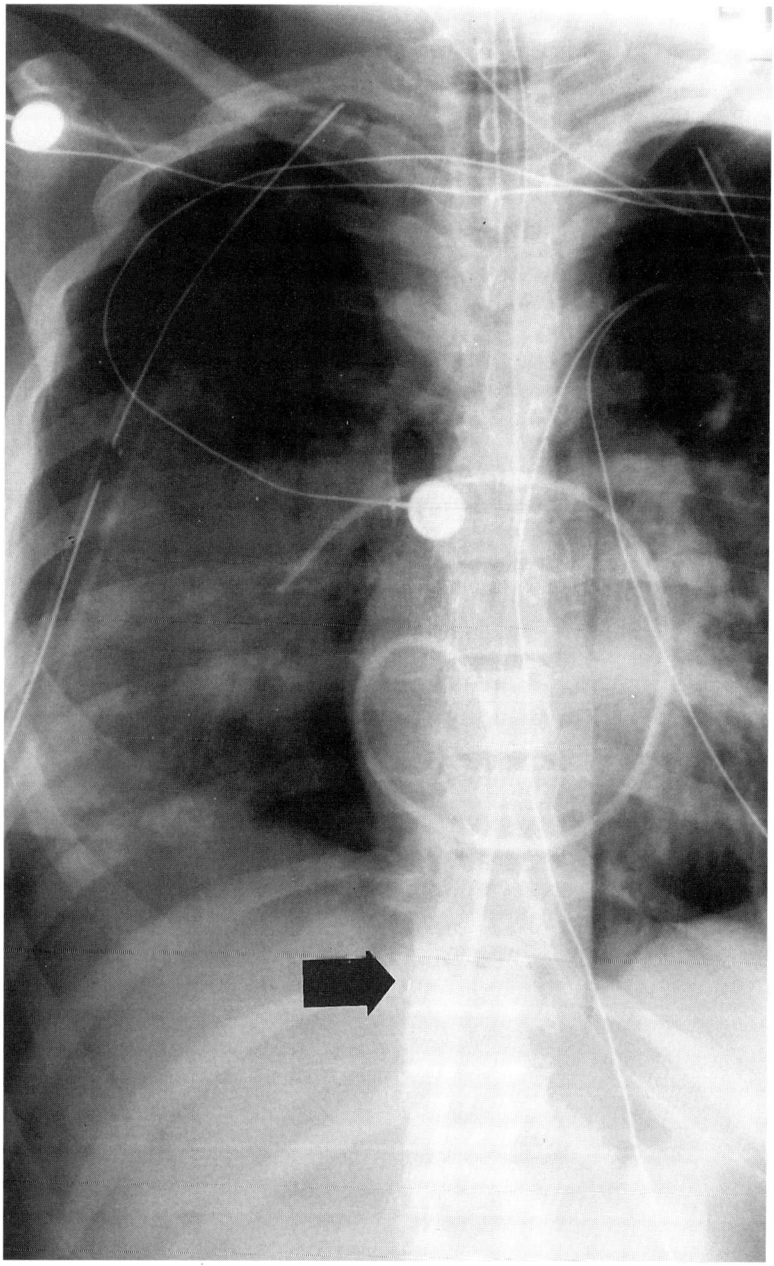

Fig. 4-23, cont'd

lateral view there would be a slightly forward position of the body of the vertebrae and the appearance of locked facets. The facets may be locked unilaterally or bilaterally. Locked facets are best seen on the AP radiograph.

Clinical Findings

Most patients with a spinal injury suffer from spinal shock. The signs of spinal shock include paralysis, loss of sensation below the level of injury, and bowel and bladder dysfunction. If the patient's injury is above the level of T6, neurogenic shock may also be present, which manifests itself by hypotension and bradycardia. In an incomplete injury, the patient will have sensory sparing and various motor losses. The patient may complain of pain over the injured vertebra.

Radiologic Appearance

The standard radiographs taken in the emergency room are AP and lateral films of the cervical spine. In order to view the seventh cervical vertebrae, it may be necessary for the nurse to pull the shoulders down. For a "swimmer's view," the patient's arm is along the head as if swimming the crawl. The x-ray beam shoots laterally across the vertebrae. Although a lateral view of the cervical spine is only 85% accurate in diagnosing injuries, it is an important first step. Oblique and pillar view radiographs may be needed to improve the view of the pedicles. Open-mouth views of the odontoid process are important to locate instability of the C1 and C2 vertebrae (Marshall et al, 1990).

Flexion-extension films are useful in evaluating a patient for spinal injury. These films must be taken under the direct supervision of a physician and only performed on patients who are awake and able to cooperate and tell the physician if and when pain occurs (Marshall et al, 1990).

Tomography can be a useful tool in identifying injuries to the cervical-thoracic junction and the thoracolumbar spine. Tomograms provide views of areas that are poorly recognizable in radiographs. They define in greater detail any bone fragments protruding into the spinal canal and facets.

CT scans can be a useful adjunct in the diagnosis of spinal injuries. With or without contrast, the scan provides a great deal of information on spinal column stability. When combined with a myelogram, CT scans give the most accurate diagnosis of the extent of the injury.

Nursing Implications

Maintaining neurologic function is the prime concern during and after diagnostic testing. Proper immobilization with a hard cervical collar and a backboard is important. Patient movement should be minimized during the diagnostic phase of care. An assessment of motor and sensory function at the time of admission and frequently during the first few days will give the nurse important information about the state of the neurologic dysfunction. Once the diagnosis of injury has been confirmed, traction or a combination of surgery and traction will be applied.

BRAIN TUMOR

Definition

Brain tumors are an overgrowth of cells that form a space-occupying lesion. The annual incidence of tumors of the brain is about 17,000 primary tumors and 17,000 metastatic tumors from other cancer sources. The incidence of tumors in men is slightly higher than in women; they affect all age groups (Hickey, 1992). Brain tumors may be benign or malignant based on the cell type. Table 4-4 describes the histological classification of the major tumors of the brain.

Pituitary tumors, which arise primarily in the anterior lobe of the pituitary gland, can be classified by grade of sella turcica enlargement and/or erosion (Adams and Victor, 1981).

Grade I — sella normal, floor may be indented
Grade II — invasive adenoma, erosion of floor
Grade III — entire floor diffusely eroded

Clinical Findings

The patient's symptoms may be vague because of the size and location of the lesion. Headache may be the patient's only symptom, or the patient may present in a coma. If the patient has a pituitary tumor, the symptoms will be related to under- or over-secretion of the pituitary hormones. Neurologic deficits correspond to the area of the brain involved.

Table 4-4 Types of brain tumors

Type of tumor	Description
COMMON BRAIN TUMORS	
Astrocytoma (Grades I and II); constitutes 25% to 30% of all cerebral gliomas	Grade I: well-defined cells Grade II: cell differentiation is less defined
Glioblastoma multiforme (also known as astrocytoma, grades III and IV); constitutes 20% of all intracranial tumors and 55% of all gliomas	Malignant, rapidly growing Composed of heterogenous cells (reflects frequent clinical progression from a slow- to rapid-growing tumor); necrotic area with multiple cysts and hemorrhagic areas within tumor; cystic tumor; slow-growing tumor; considered benign if completely excised
Astrocytoma of the cerebellum (Grades I to IV); a childhood tumor	
Astrocytoma of the optic nerves and chiasma (spongioblastoma); most common in children	As the tumor grows, it enlarges the optic foramen with little distortion of the surrounding structures Slow-growing tumor
Ependymoma (grades I to IV); a tumor commonly found in children and young adults; more benign form may be called astroblastoma; more malignant form may be called ependymoblastoma	A glioma arising from the lining of the ventricles Slow-growing tumor
Oligodendroglioma (grades I to IV)	Calcification noted on radiological examination in about 50% of patients Slow-growing tumor
Mixed gliomas; may be names for the predominant tumor cell present	Composed histologically of two or more cell types of astrocytoma/glioblastoma, oligodendroglioma, or ependymoma in any combination

Table 4-4 Types of brain tumors—cont'd

Type of tumor	Description
Medulloblastoma; a childhood tumor	Rapidly growing tumor that can obstruct CSF flow Seeding into the third and lateral ventricles, as well as the cisterna magna and along the spinal cord, is common
Meningioma	Firm, encapsulated tumor arising from arachnoid granulations/meninges Slow-growing tumor that can become large before symptoms appear Causes compression of the brain
Metastic brain tumors	Ten percent of all brain tumors are metastatic from other parts of the body (lungs, breast, stomach, lower GI tract, pancreas, and kidney) Spread to the brain by blood Usually well-differentiated from the rest of the brain
Acoustic neuroma (schwannoma)	Arises from the sheath of Schwann cells Sizes varies from the size of a pea to that of a walnut Considered a benign tumor, but located in an area that is often inaccessible Bilateral tumors are occasionally found Slow-growing tumor Tumor may entwine other cranial nerves that would cause severe deficits if the tumor was completely excised Bilateral tumors are possible; when they occur, they are due to a hereditary problem of chromosome 22; the tumors are part of central neurofibromatosis
Chordoma	Arises from remnants of the embryonic notochord May appear as a cerebellopontine angle tumor Affects males more frequently than females Occurs in patients in their 30s and 40s

Table 4-4 Types of brain tumors—cont'd

Type of tumor	Description
PITUITARY TUMORS	
Pituitary adenomas	Classified by the type of hormone(s) secreted: prolactin-secreting (6% to 70% of all tumors in males and females); growth hormone-secreting (10% to 15% of all tumors); ACTH secreting Classified by function: nonfunctioning—produce symptoms as a result of pressure on adjacent structures (e.g., optic nerves, bitemporal hemianopia); functioning (or hormone-secreting)—cause endocrine syndromes (e.g., Cushing's hyperprolactinemia, acromegaly). Classified by grade of sella turcica enlargement and/or erosion: Enclosed adenomas: I—sella normal, floor may be indented; II—sella enlarged, floor intact; III—invasive adenomas, localized erosion of the floor; IV—entire floor diffusely eroded Classified by suprasellar extension (Hardy) A—no suprasellar extension; B—suprasellar bulge does not reach the floor of the 3rd ventricle; C—tumor reaches the 3rd ventricle, distorting chiasmatic recess; D—tumor fills the 3rd ventricle almost to the foramen of Monro
DEVELOPMENTAL TUMORS	
Craniopharyngioma	Thought to arise from Rathke's pouch Solid cystic tumors Can compress the pituitary and may even amputate the pituitary stalk Approximately 75% have calcified areas Tumor growth is directed upward, resulting in invagination of the third ventricle and possible blockage of CSF flow Optic chiasm is elevated as a result of tumor, resulting in traction on optic nerves
Epidermoid and dermoid cysts	Cysts of congenital origin arising from the ectodermal layer Cysts are lined with stratified squamous epithelium Epidermoid cysts contain keratin, cellular debris, and cholesterol Dermoid cysts contain hair and sebaceous glands

Radiologic Appearance

Skull films are usually taken but are of limited value in the true diagnosis of brain tumor. If the tumor is large enough to cause a midline shift of structures, the pineal gland, which is usually calcified in adults, will be skewed to the side away from the tumor. Abnormal calcification in the brain raises the suspicion of a calcified component located within a tumor. If the tumor has caused increased intracranial pressure, the skull may show signs of bone erosion and extreme thinning.

Tumors that invade the orbits of the eyes or other facial structures may or may not be observed on a radiograph. However, again the clinician may see signs of displacement of normal anatomical structures. Bone erosion may also be noted.

The most accurate way of diagnosing a brain tumor and its location is by CT scan. The CT scan can differentiate the type of lesion the patient has, e.g., abscess, cysts, or hydrocephalus. It can even suggest a primary tumor from a metastatic lesion. The scan precisely locates the tumor and describes the size. Contrast media can be injected to better demonstrate the tumor (Fig. 4-24). The tumor will generally appear lighter than the surrounding brain tumor.

Occasionally a nuclear medicine brain scan will be done to diagnose a brain tumor. The tumor within the brain tissue breaks down the blood/brain barrier in the tumor bed. Normal brain scans show an even uptake of the radionucleotide injected for the scan. If the patient has a tumor, the area around the tumor bed will have a concentrated uptake that appears as a black or very dark area on the radiograph. The approximate size and location of the tumor will be described by this examination. Since the advent of CT scanning, brain scans are rarely performed.

Nursing Implications

If the patient has increased ICP, placing the patient flat for a CT scan may worsen the patient's neurologic symptoms during and after the diagnostic study. If the patient is to receive contrast, a skin test is done to ensure that the patient is not allergic to the dye (Hickey, 1992). If contrast media is used, the patient usually receives nothing by mouth for 4 to 8 hours before the CT. The patient may require sedation to minimize movement during the scan. The patient requires no special care after the scan. If contrast media is given, the patient should be kept well hydrated.

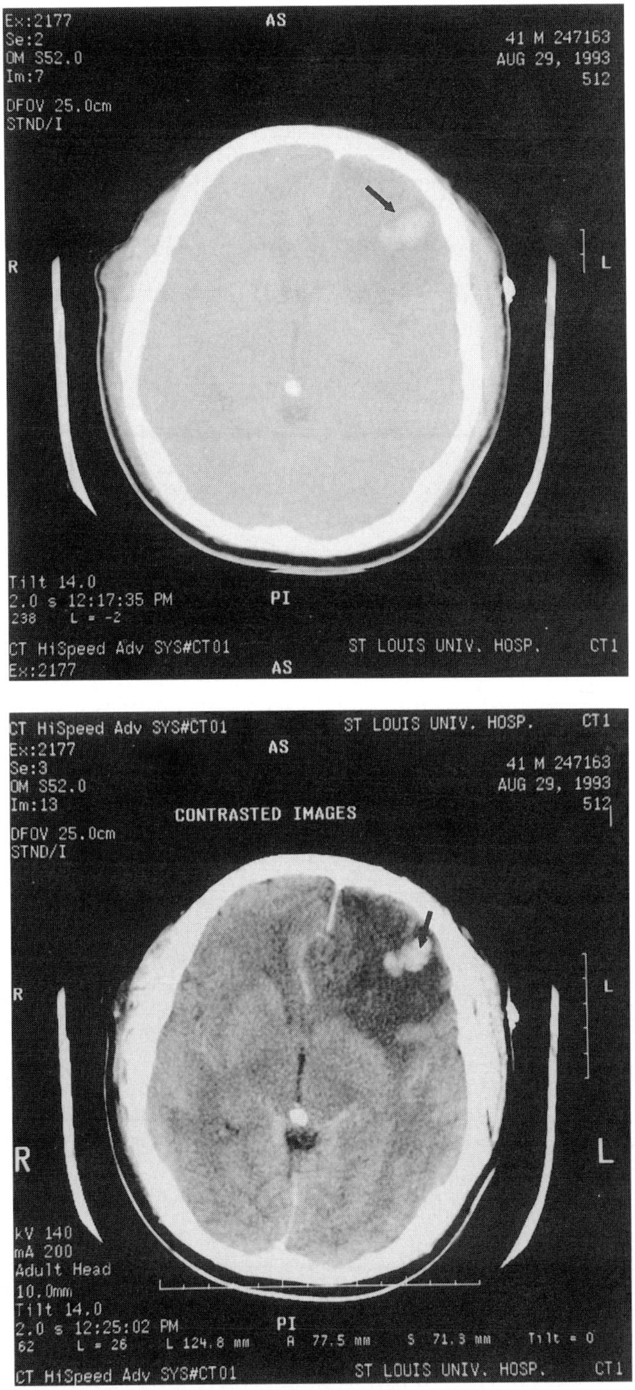

A

B

Fig. 4-24 **A** through **F,** Cranial tumor. The brain windows of this CT scan demonstrate large bilateral tumors with a slight mass effect.

Continued.

C

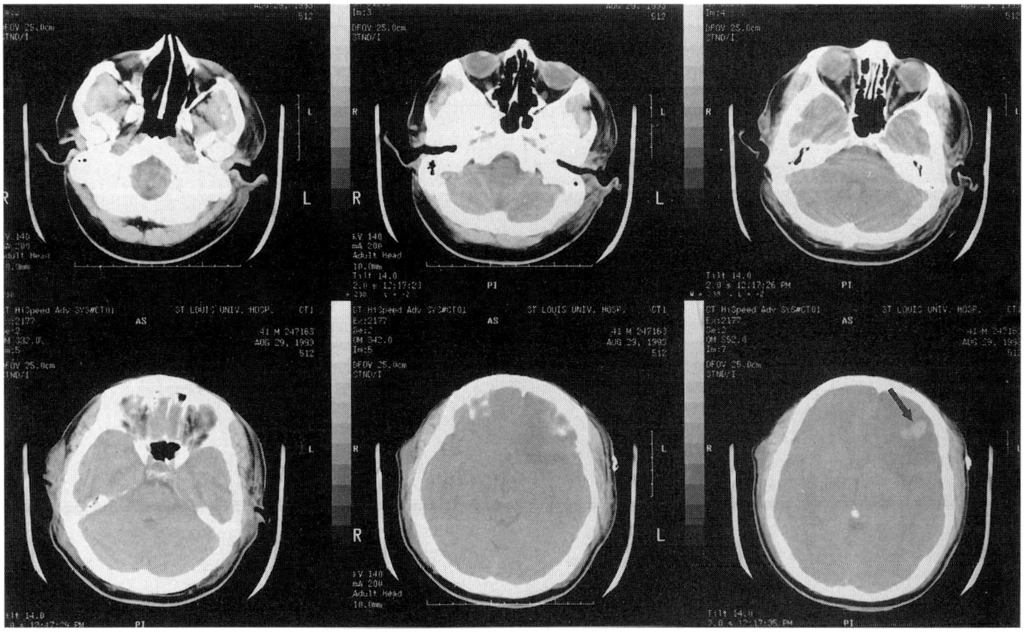

D

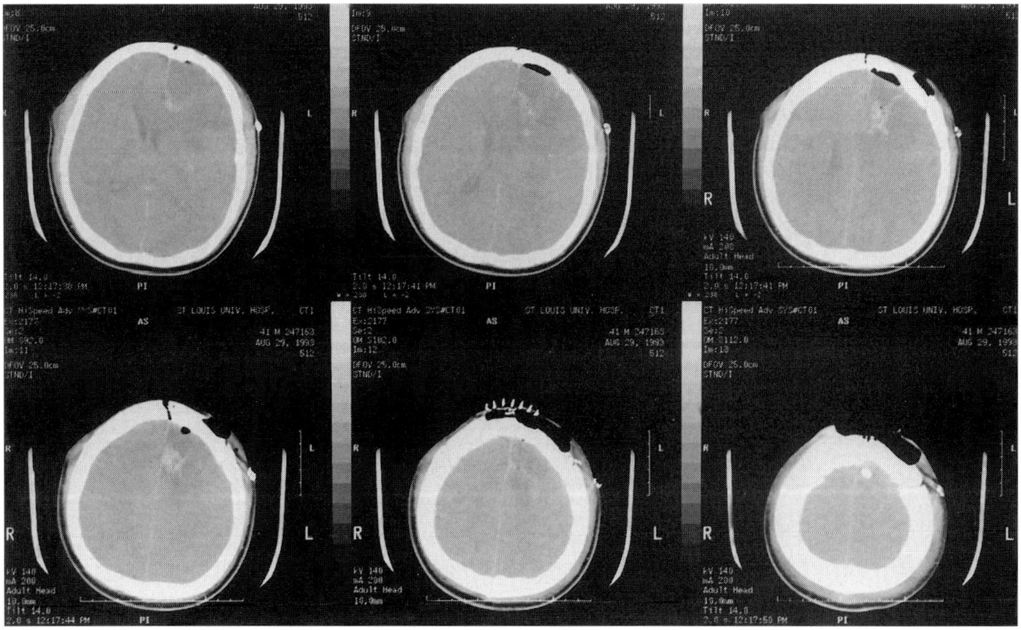

Fig. 4-24, cont'd

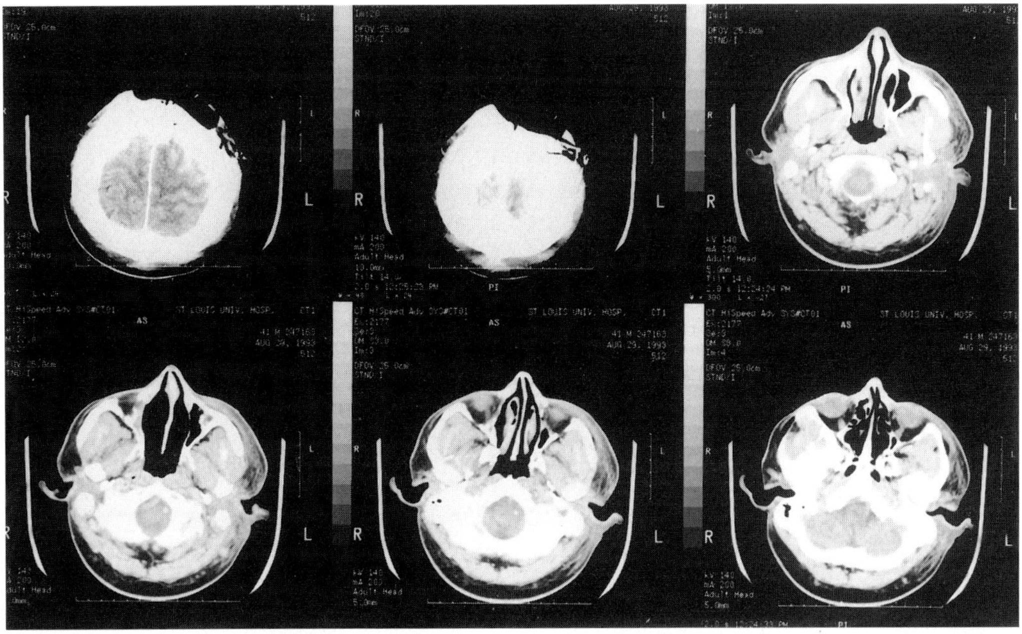

E

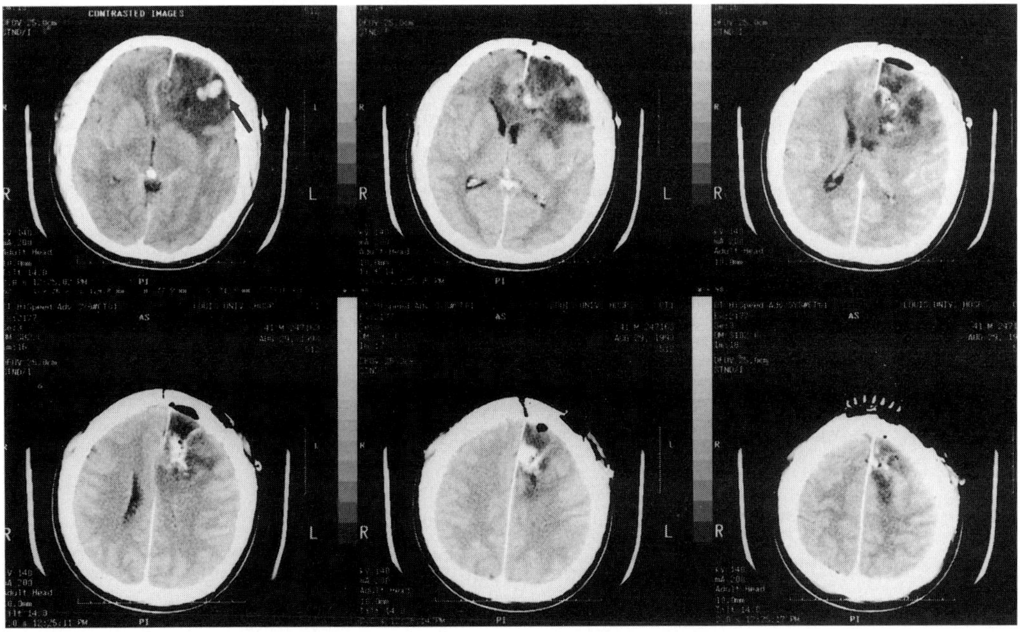

F

Fig. 4-24, cont'd

SPINAL CORD TUMOR

Definition

Spinal cord tumors are an abnormal collection of cells in or compressing the cord. The incidence of spinal cord tumors is much less than that of brain tumors: approximately 0.5% to 1% of all tumors. Spinal tumors occur equally in males and females and are rare in children under 10 years of age. Primary tumors make up 70% of all spinal tumors arising from the epidural vessels, spinal meninges, or the glial element (Adams and Victor, 1981).

Spinal tumors are classified as extramedullary (outside of the spinal cord) or intramedullary (within the cord). Extramedullary tumors may be extradural or intradural.

Clinical Findings

Depending on the type of tumor and extent of involvement, the patient's symptoms vary from back pain to complete paralysis below the lesion. Paresthesias and other sensory changes may also occur.

Radiologic Appearance

The x-ray film of the vertebral column is rarely helpful in diagnosing a spinal cord tumor. If the tumor has invaded the bone, increased density of the affected vertebra or vertebrae may be seen. Degeneration of the vertebral body caused by the tumor will also be apparent on the film.

The myelogram has become the mainstay for diagnosing spinal cord tumors. Contrast medium is injected into the subarachnoid space, and x-ray films are taken of the spinal cord and vertebral column. A tumor that obstructs the flow of contrast media will be apparent on the films. If the tumor is intramedullary, the spinal cord will appear widened and the subarachnoid space will appear narrowed (Hickey, 1992) (Fig. 4-25).

Nursing Implications

The patient who has a CT myelogram will be tilted with his or her head down to allow the contrast medium to cover the entire subarachnoid space. The patient will have to lie flat, which may increase his or her pain.

Patient management after the myelogram depends on the type of contrast media used: oil-based or water-soluble. If the patient is to receive an oil-based

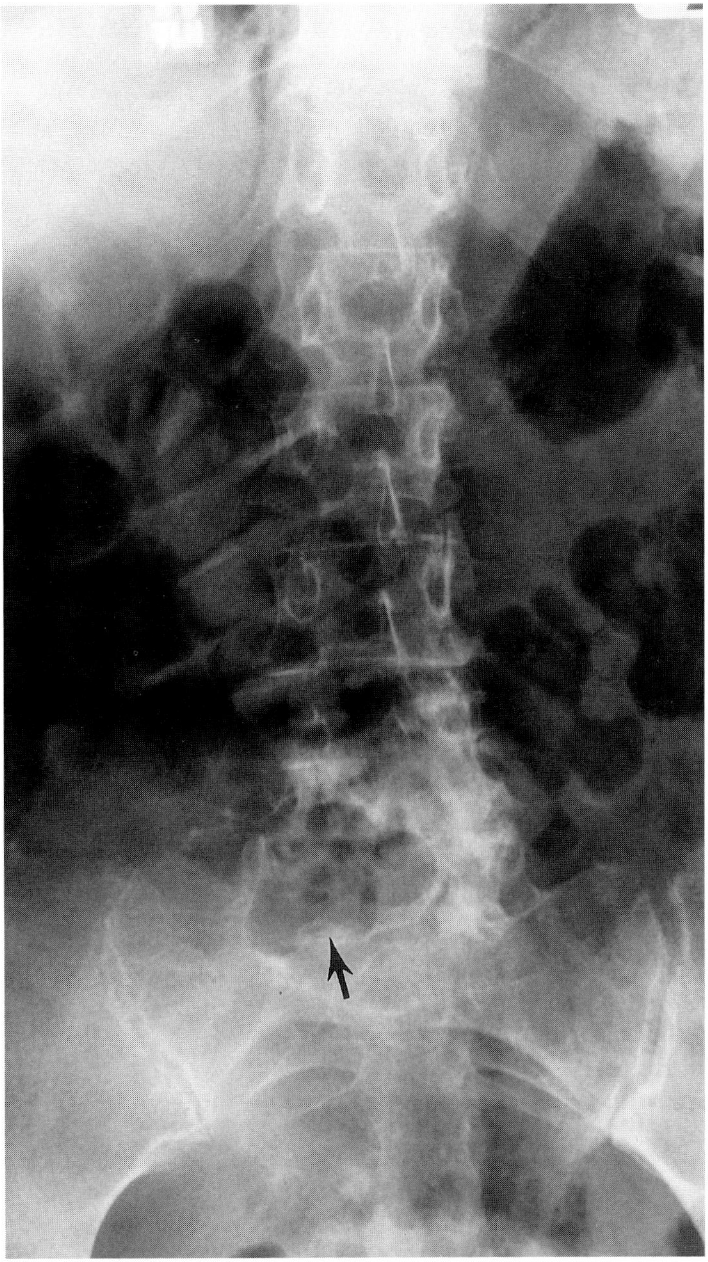

A

Fig. 4-25 **A** and **B,** Spinal cord tumor. A large lower lumbar tumor involving the spinal cord and causing bony destruction was found on this radiograph. A subsequent CT scan and MRI were performed before surgery. The patient also had arthritis of the spine, as evidenced by the bright white spots in the joints.

Continued.

B

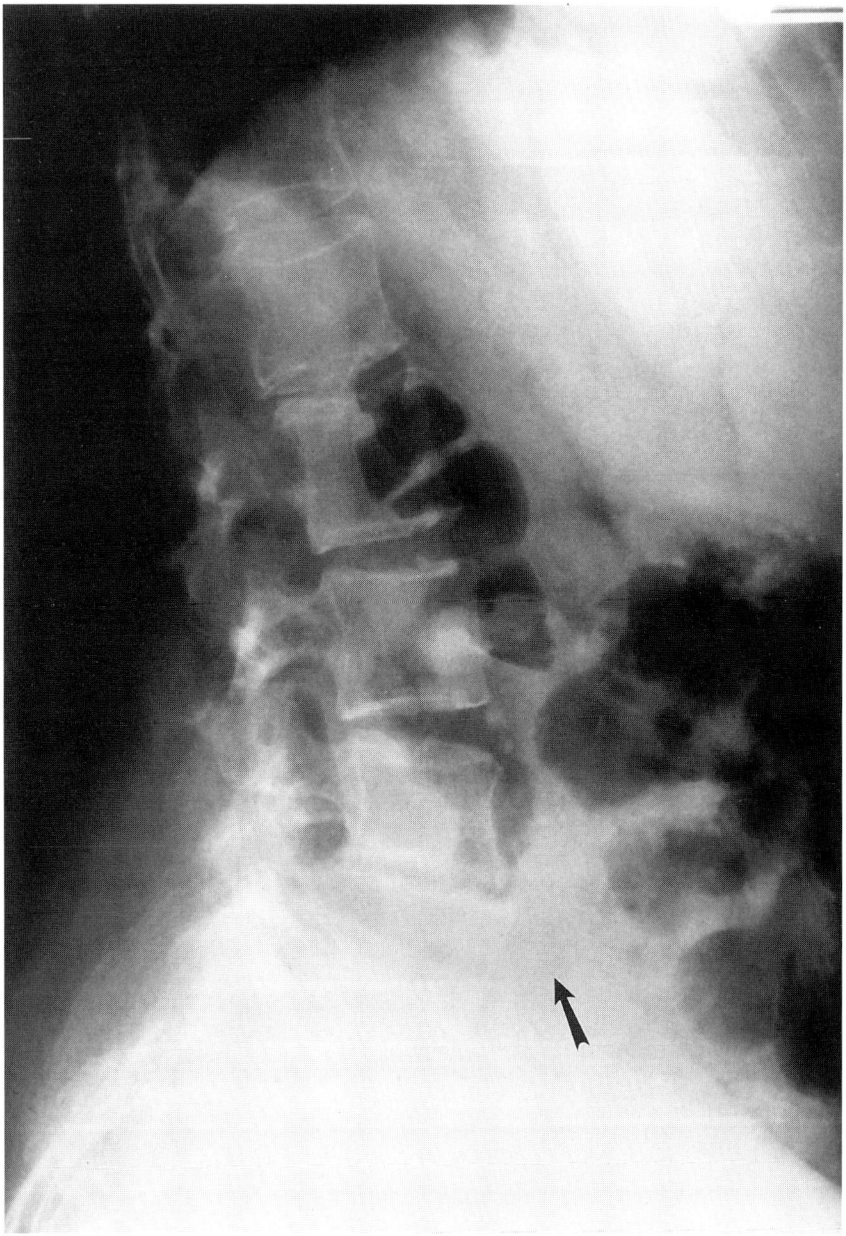

Fig. 4-25, cont'd

dye, he or she is not allowed to eat or drink before the procedure. A narcotic or sedative is generally ordered 1 hour before the test. The patient should lie flat for 4 to 8 hours after the myelogram. Forcing fluids assists the patient to clear the dye. The patient should be observed for signs of any reaction to the dye (Hickey, 1992).

The use of water-based media has become popular. Food and fluids may be consumed before the myelogram. All neuroleptic drugs, monoamine oxidase inhibitors, and psychostimulants must be discontinued 48 hours before the test. After the test the patient's head is elevated to 30 to 45 degrees for the first 12 hours. Phenothiazines are avoided and fluids are forced for at least 24 hours (Hickey, 1992).

BRAIN ABSCESS

Definition

A brain abscess is caused by a systemic infectious process or an infection that extends into the brain tissue. The major sources of infection in the brain are the middle part of the ear, the mastoid, the sinuses, and the teeth. Approximately 40% of all brain abscesses are the result of a middle ear or mastoid infection (Hickey, 1992). The location of the abscess depends on the source and the method by which the organism spreads.

Clinical Findings

Initially the patient may complain of headache, malaise, fever, confusion, drowsiness, and seizures (focal or generalized). If the abscess continues to enlarge, the patient will become stuporous or comatose and may develop increased ICP. The neurologic deficits will vary according to the location of the abscess.

Radiologic Appearance

On the CT scan, the brain abscess has a very characteristic appearance—it is surrounded by a white ring. This ring distinguishes the abscess from a tumor when contrast medium is used (Fig. 4-26).

A

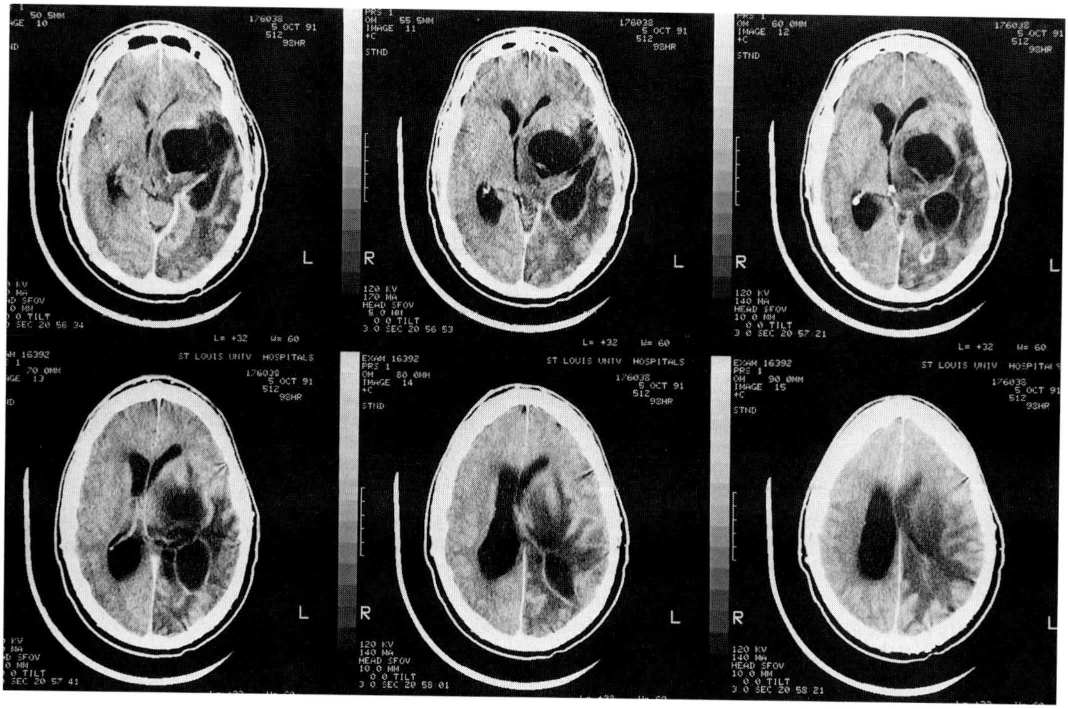

Fig. 4-26 **A** and **B,** Brain abscess. Multiple, loculated, "white" rim-enhancing lesions in the brain windows as viewed on a CT scan. Note the significant left-to-right midline shift and abnormal ventricular configurations.

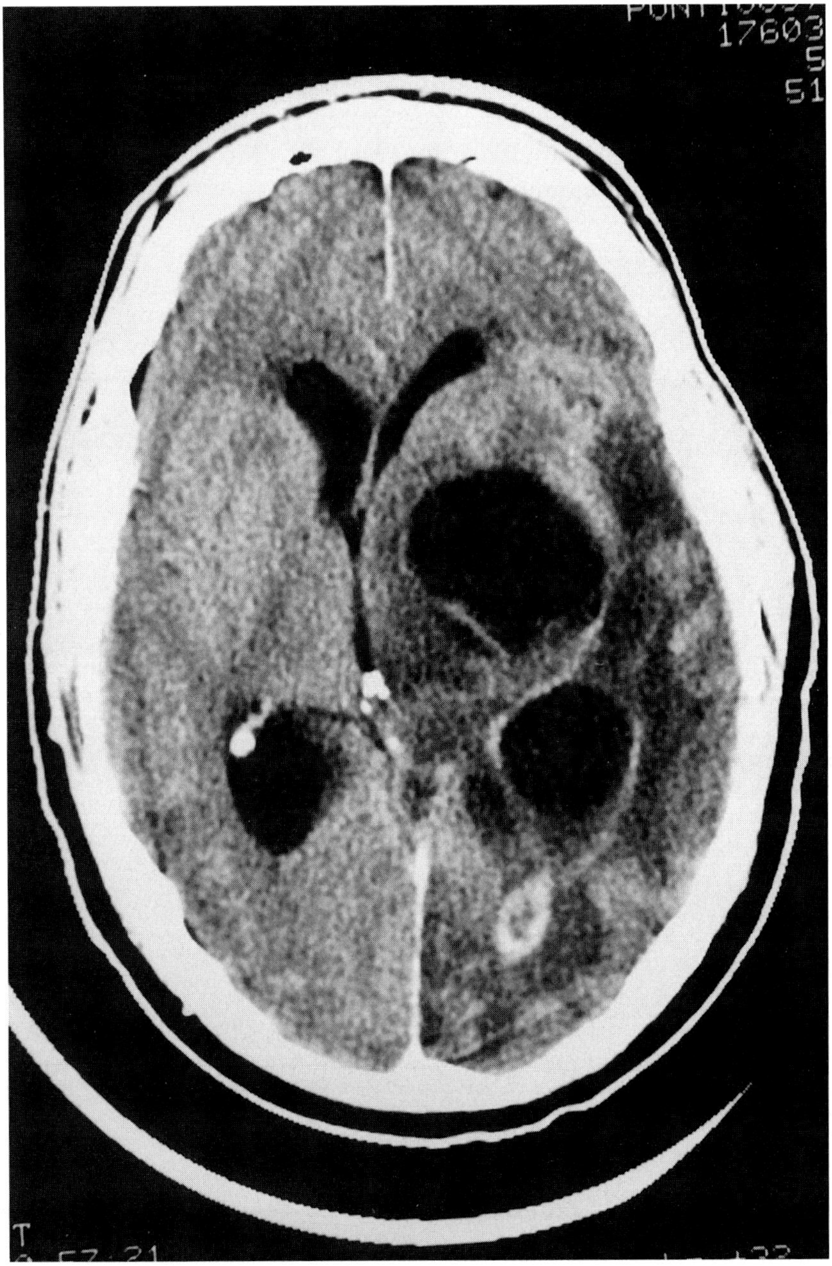

B

Fig. 4-26, cont'd

Nursing Implications

The patient will be positioned flat for a CT scan, which may increase the patient's neurologic deficits and raise the ICP. If the patient has a severe headache, lying flat may worsen the pain. Frequent neurologic assessment is important in patients with brain abscesses. Monitoring of other infections must be incorporated into the patient's care.

TEST YOURSELF

Use your knowledge of assessing a neurological radiograph to answer the question under Fig. 4-27.

A

B

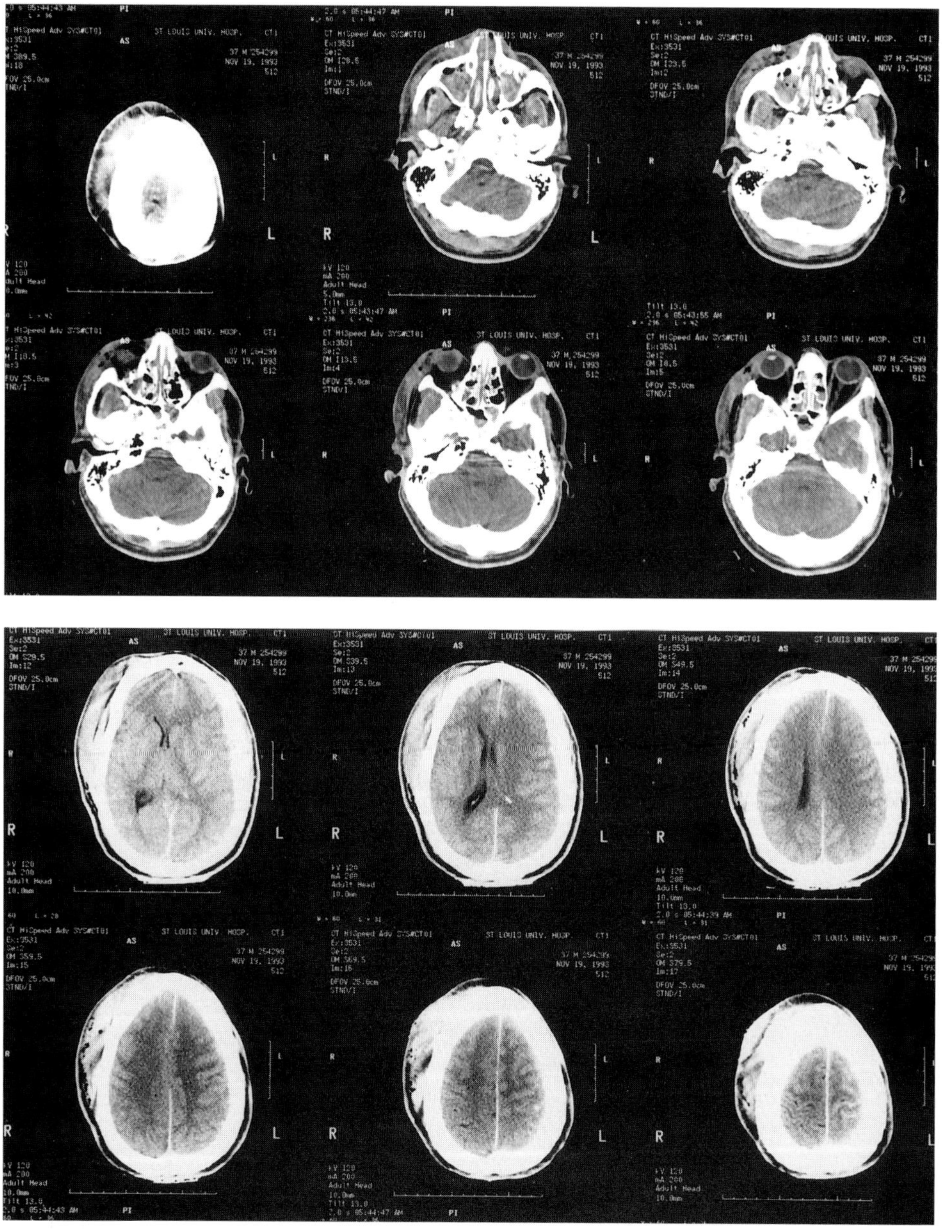

Fig. 4-27 What abnormalities are present in the bone and brain windows that would warrant specialized nursing care?

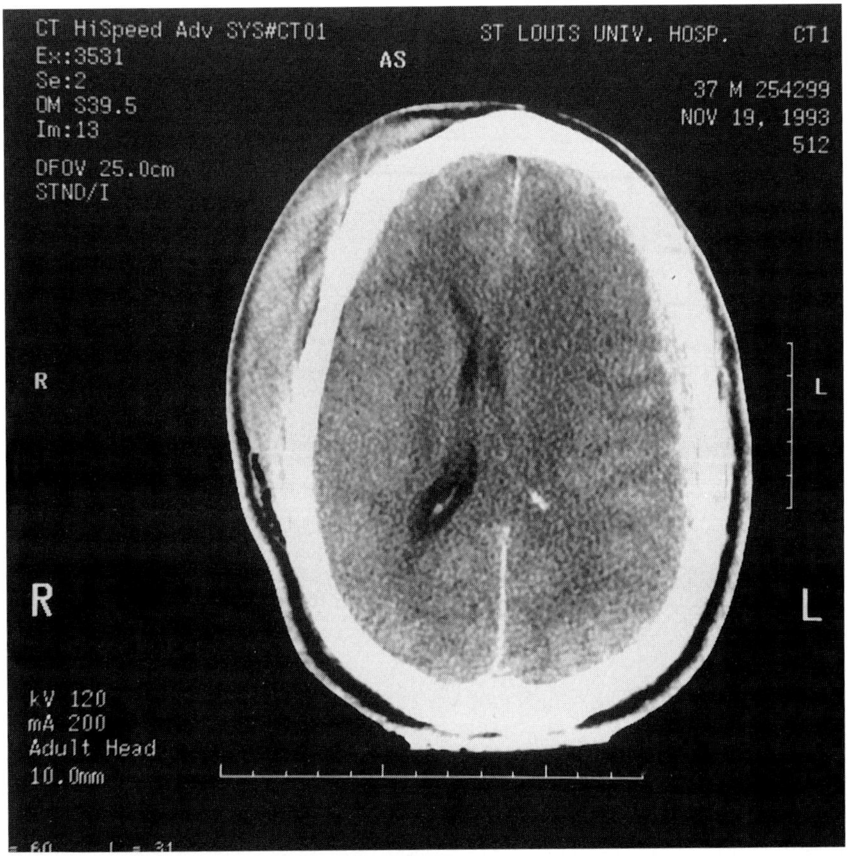

C

Fig. 4-27, cont'd

REFERENCES

Adams R, Victor M: *Principles of Neurology,* ed 2, New York, 1991, McGraw-Hill.
Deli SL, Bower TC: Maxillofacial and soft tissue injuries. In Cardona V et al, editors: *Trauma Nursing: From Resuscitation through Rehabilitation.* Philadelphia, 1988, WB Saunders.
Hickey JV: *Neurological and Neurosurgical Nursing:* ed 3, Philadelphia, 1992, JB Lippincott.
Marshall SB et al: *Neuroscience Critical Care,* Philadelphia, 1990, WB Saunders.
President's Commission for the Study of Ethical Problems in Medicine and Biomedical Behavioral Research, Washington, DC, 1981, U.S. Government Printing Office.
Tessler P: Experimental study of fractures of the upper jaw (translated from LeForte R: Etude experimentelle sui les fractures de la machoir superiem. Rev Chir 23:479, 1901). In McDowell F, editor: *The Source Book of Plastic and Reconstructive Surgery,* Baltimore, 1977, Williams and Wilkins.

5 Assessment of the Patient
Abdominal Radiography

The purpose of this chapter is to review pertinent anatomy and physiology of the abdomen for the purpose of assessing abdominal radiographs. The most common findings seen on abdominal radiographs of critically ill patients are presented.

The abdomen is located between the diaphragm and the pelvis. The abdomen contains a seromembranous peritoneal lining, which is similar to the pleura in the chest cavity. The peritoneal lining or sac has two portions: the parietal or outer layer, which adheres to the abdominal wall, diaphragm, and pelvis, and the visceral or inner layer, which adheres to the abdominal organs. The narrow space between the two linings is called the *peritoneal cavity*. The peritoneal cavity allows pelvic and thoracic surgery to be performed without invasion into the abdomen or chest, respectively.

An ideal examination of the abdomen allows time for the evacuation of fecal material and gas. In the critically ill patient this is often not possible. With a patient who is not acutely ill, dietary modifications, laxatives, or enemas may be needed to evacuate the bowel to optimize examination of the various organs. Bowel preparation is not performed in patients with suspected intestinal obstruction, perforation, or visceral rupture.

The most commonly performed examination of the abdomen is the anterior to posterior supine "flat plate" or "KUB" (*k*idneys, *u*reter, *b*ladder radiograph). The patient may also be positioned upright or in a lateral decubitus position, allowing free air or fluid levels to be identified by the examiner. The traditional obstructive or acute abdominal series includes a flat plate, an upright, and a chest radiograph. It is often important for the nurse to shield the patient's gonads during radiologic procedures involving the abdomen.

For the purpose of radiographic assessment, the abdomen is usually divided into four quadrants (right and left, upper and lower) that intersect at the umbilicus. Some radiologists may use nine regions (right and left superior hypochondrium and epigastrium, right and left middle lumbar and umbilical, right and left inferior iliac and hypogastrium). Also assessed when examining the abdominal (digestive) systems is the esophagus, most of which is better viewed on the chest radiograph. A chest radiograph is often part of an upper abdominal series.

In the right upper quadrant the main organ visualized is the liver, although special techniques can image the bile-secreting gallbladder and the right kidney (Fig. 5-1). The liver, which sits just under the right diaphragm, measures approximately 8.5 inches (21.5 cm) at the widest point and 6.5 inches (16.5 cm) at the longest point. The liver is anatomically divided into two major and two minor lobes; the latter contain the hilar area called the *porta.* The hepatic artery, portal vein, and hepatic bile ducts are located in the porta. The posterior hepatic veins empty into the inferior vena cava of the heart.

The stomach and spleen are in the left upper quadrant. The stomach is a sac that connects the esophagus and the small intestine. The stomach has an anterior and a posterior surface. The right border of the stomach is called the *lesser curvature;* it begins at the esophagus and ends at the small intestine. The *greater curvature* of the stomach, located on the left and inferior sides of the stomach, is 4 to 5 times longer than the lesser curvature. The stomach is divided into four parts: the cardia, which surrounds the esophagus; the fundus, which is the top of the stomach and abuts the dome of the left diaphragm; the body, which is the main portion of the stomach; and the pylorus, which is the distal portion of the stomach. The bean-shaped spleen is about 5 inches long and 3 inches wide. It is located laterally just behind the stomach and below the diaphragm. Also in this area are the left kidney and the pancreas.

The small intestine (bowel) and large intestine (colon) occupy the lower quadrants. The small bowel, which is about 22 feet long and 1 to 1.5 inches (2 to 3 cm) wide, extends from the pyloric sphincter of the stomach to the ileocecal valve and first crosses the abdomen from left to right. The small bowel has three portions: the duodenum, jejunum, and ileum. The duodenum makes up the first 8 to 10 inches of the small bowel and has the appearance of a C. Radiologists designate four portions of the jejunum for radiographic assessment: first (superior) about 2 inches, second (descending) about 3 to 4 inches, third (inferior or horizontal) about 2.5 inches, and fourth (ascending) about 2.5 inches (Ballinger, 1991). The duodenum joins the jejunum at a sharp curve in the digestive tract. The remainder of the small bowel is divided into the jejunum (⅖ of its length) and ileum (approximately ⅗ of its length). The

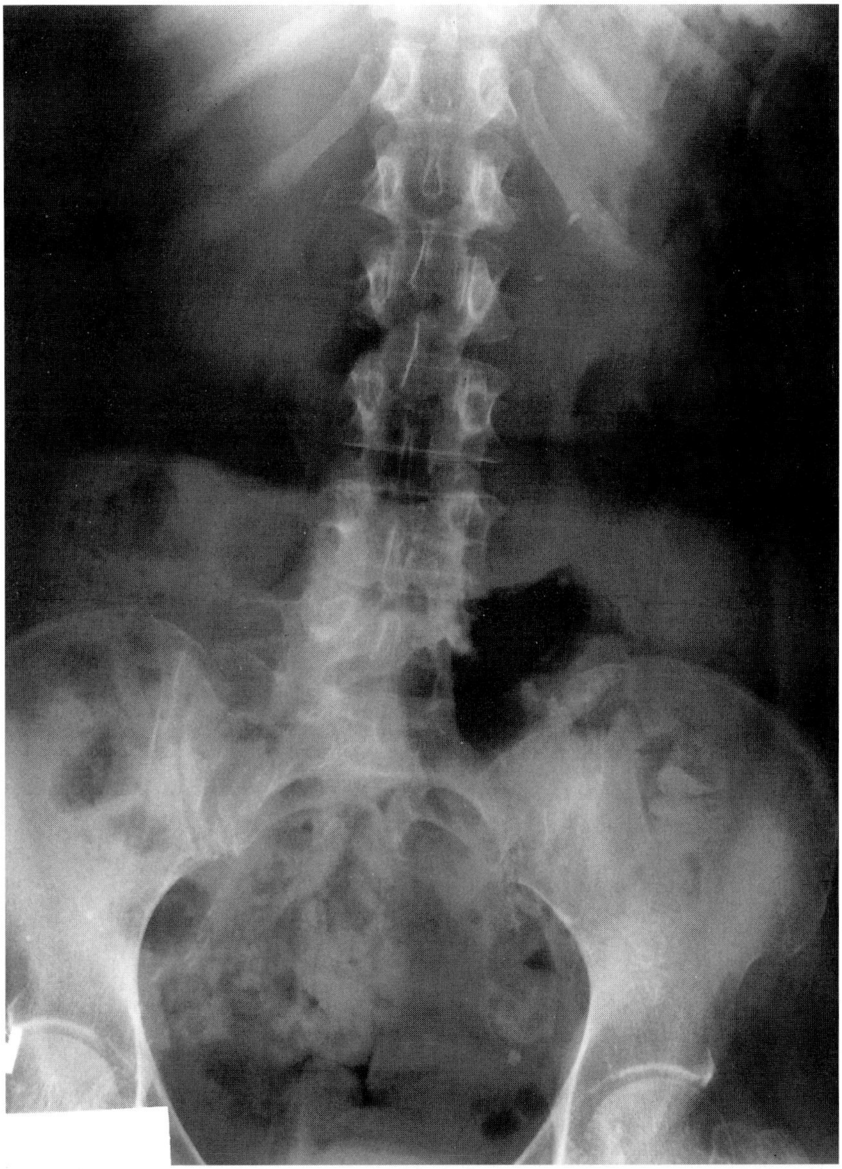

A

Fig. 5-1 **A** and **B,** Normal structures on an abdominal radiograph.

Continued.

B

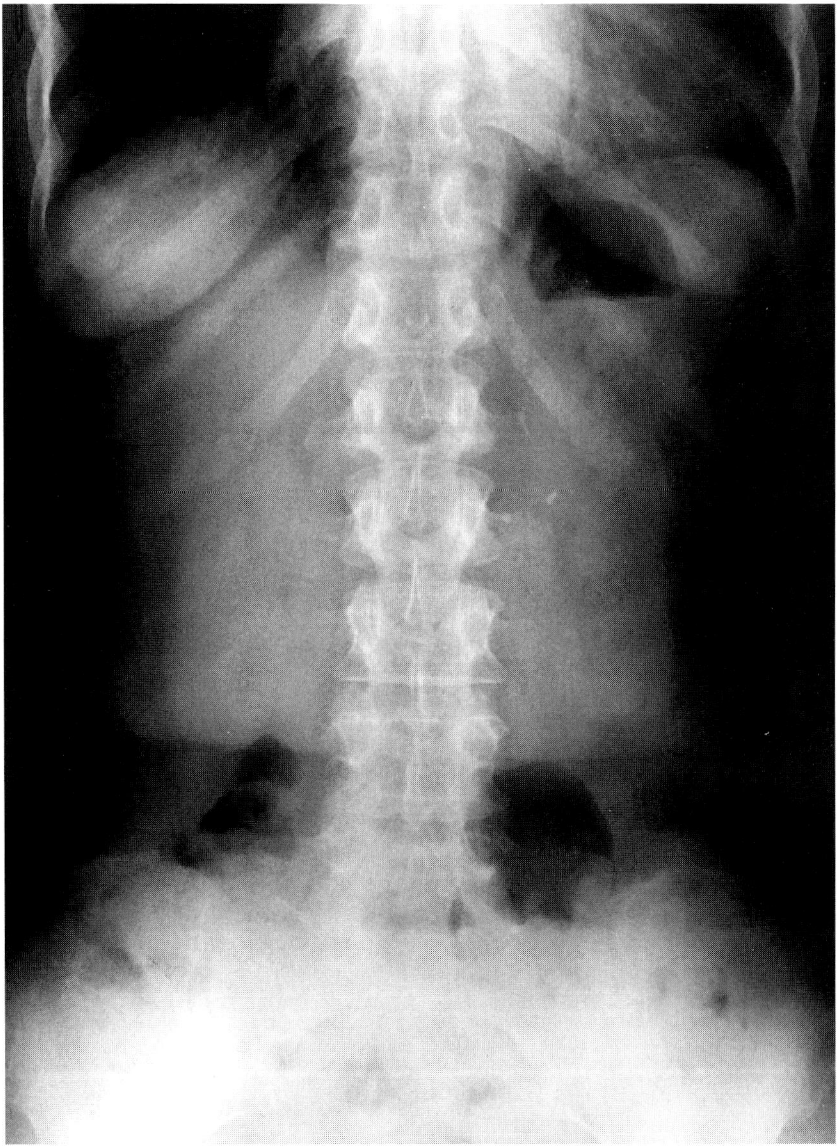

Fig. 5-1, cont'd

distal portion of the small bowel empties into the colon in the right lower quadrant. The colon then ascends and crosses from right to left like an arch before it ends in the midline sigmoid colon and rectum. The four portions of the colon are the ascending, transverse, descending, and sigmoid portions. The colon contains bands of muscles that form pouches or sacculations called *haustra*. Haustra are easy to see on an abdominal radiograph. Common findings on abdominal radiographs follow.

GASTRIC AIR BUBBLE

Definition

A gastric air bubble is a common finding in abdominal and chest radiographs, especially if the examination was performed with the patient in an upright position. A gastric air bubble is helpful in determining the presence of a pleural effusion and correct position of nasogastric tubes.

Clinical Findings

Because a gastric air bubble is normal, there are no specific findings. If the patient has swallowed large amounts of air, the nurse should be able to percuss hyperresonance or tympany over the stomach. If there is a large gastric air bubble, the nurse may also observe an enlarged upper abdomen.

Radiologic Appearance

A gastric air bubble usually appears on the left side of the chest in the fundus of the stomach. Only a few millimeters of space should separate the gastric air bubble from the diaphragm. The gastric air bubble is usually about the size of a golf ball. If it is larger, there may be outlet obstruction or the patient may have swallowed large amounts of air, such as occurs during cardiopulmonary resuscitation (Fig. 5-2).

Nursing Implications

If the gastric air bubble appears unusually large, the patient may require a nasogastric tube or repositioning of an existing nasogastric tube to decompress the stomach.

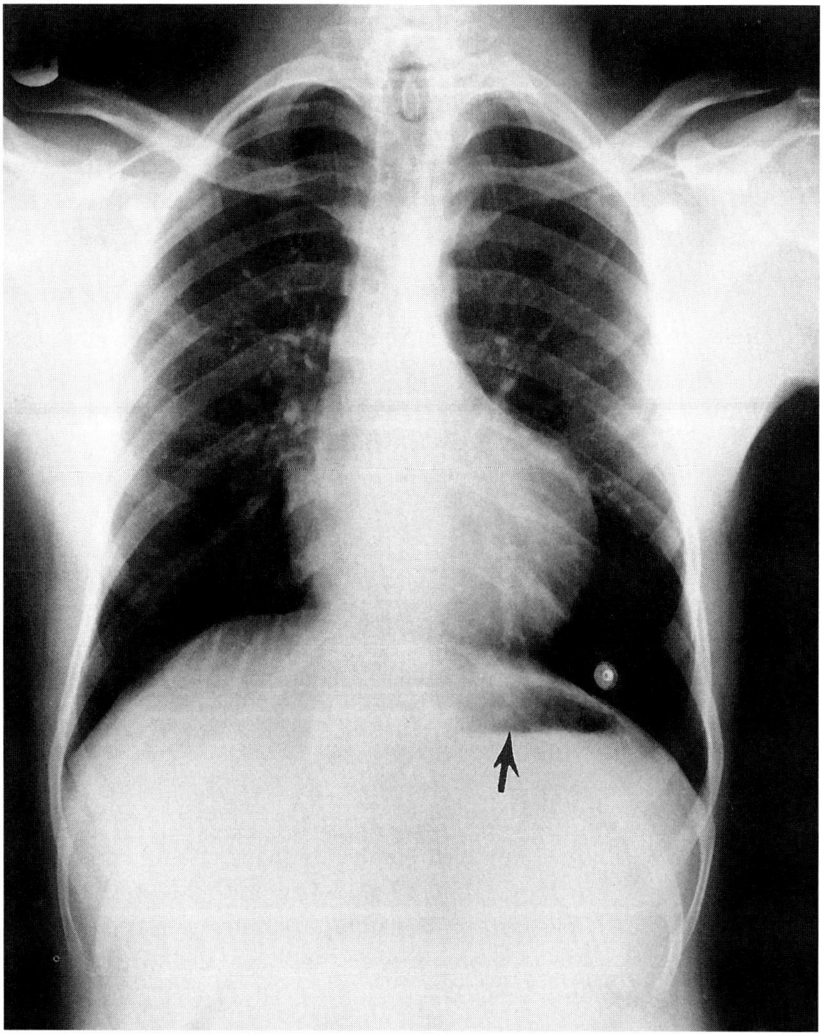

Fig. 5-2 Normal position of the gastric air bubble just under the left hemidiaphragm. The size of the gastric air bubble varies with the amount of air in the patient's stomach.

FEEDING TUBE

Definition

There are three basic types of feeding tubes. The simple nasogastric tube, such as a Levine or Salem sump, is usually of a larger diameter and delivers food into the stomach. Patients with this type of feeding tube are given bolus feedings. The smaller-bore, titanium-weighted nasogastric tube travels into the small bowel to deliver slow, continuous drip feedings. Some patients have a percutaneous gastric or small bowel feeding tube inserted for chronic or permanent enteral nutrition.

Clinical Findings

Each type of tube has a different connection system with which the nurse should become familiar. When feedings are initiated with a gastric versus small bowel tube, the nurse assesses for gastric residual of tube feedings at regular intervals throughout the day. The nurse should also routinely assess the amount of tubing that extends from the nare. Some patients may have a nasogastric tube for drainage and a titanium-weighted feeding tube (see the discussion of nasogastric tubes).

Radiologic Appearance

If there are no feedings in the feeding tube, only a thin radiopaque line is evident on the radiograph. When feedings are in the tube, the radiopaque line may be obscured by the wider (2 to 3 mm) fluid density of the tube. A nasogastric feeding tube is in the correct position when the tip of the tube is in the lower portion of the stomach near the fundus. The tip of the tube should not be in the lung or the esophagus. The tip of the titanium-weighted feeding tube is easy to locate on an x-ray film because the metallic-density tip is approximately 2 inches in length. Although there is some variability among clinicians, the correct position of this type of feeding tube is in the small bowel, usually in the distal duodenum or jejunum. Rarely the nurse will observe kinking or looping of the tube in the stomach or small bowel (Figs. 5-3, 5-4, and 5-5).

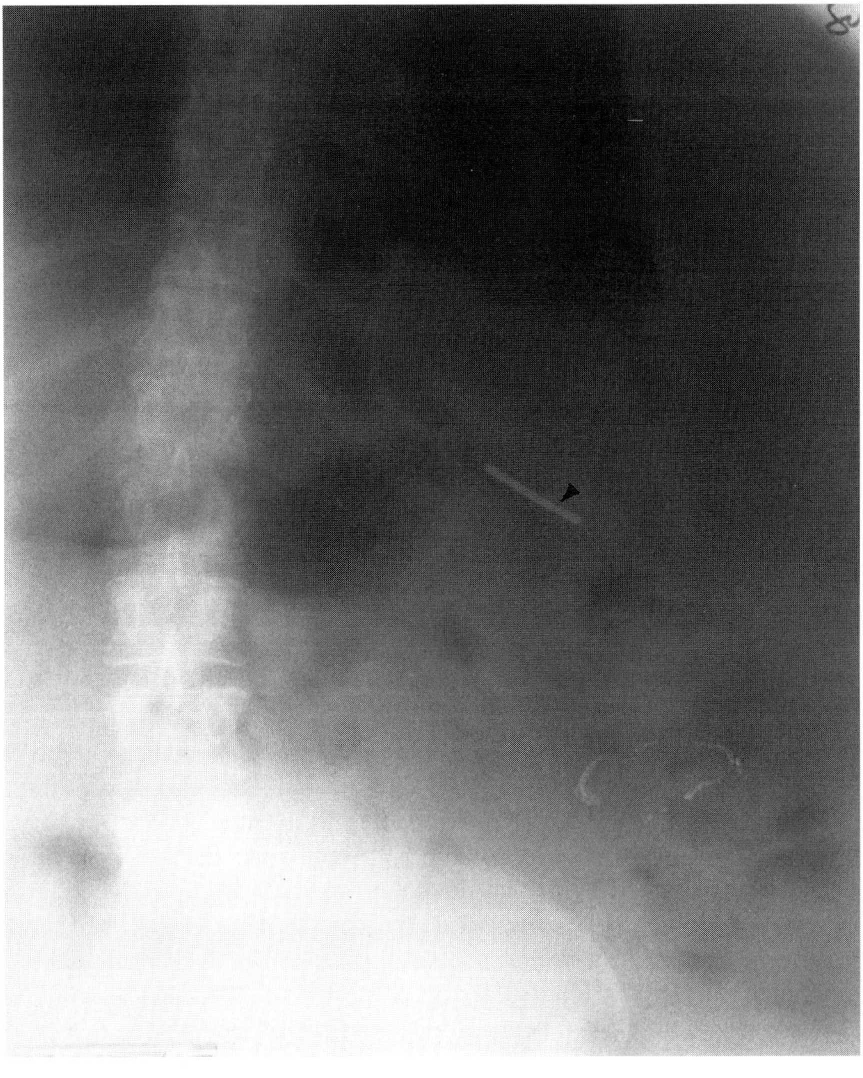

Fig. 5-3 Locate the tip of the nasogastric tube in the stomach. Notice that the tip of the tube lies in the lower portion of the stomach near the pylorus.

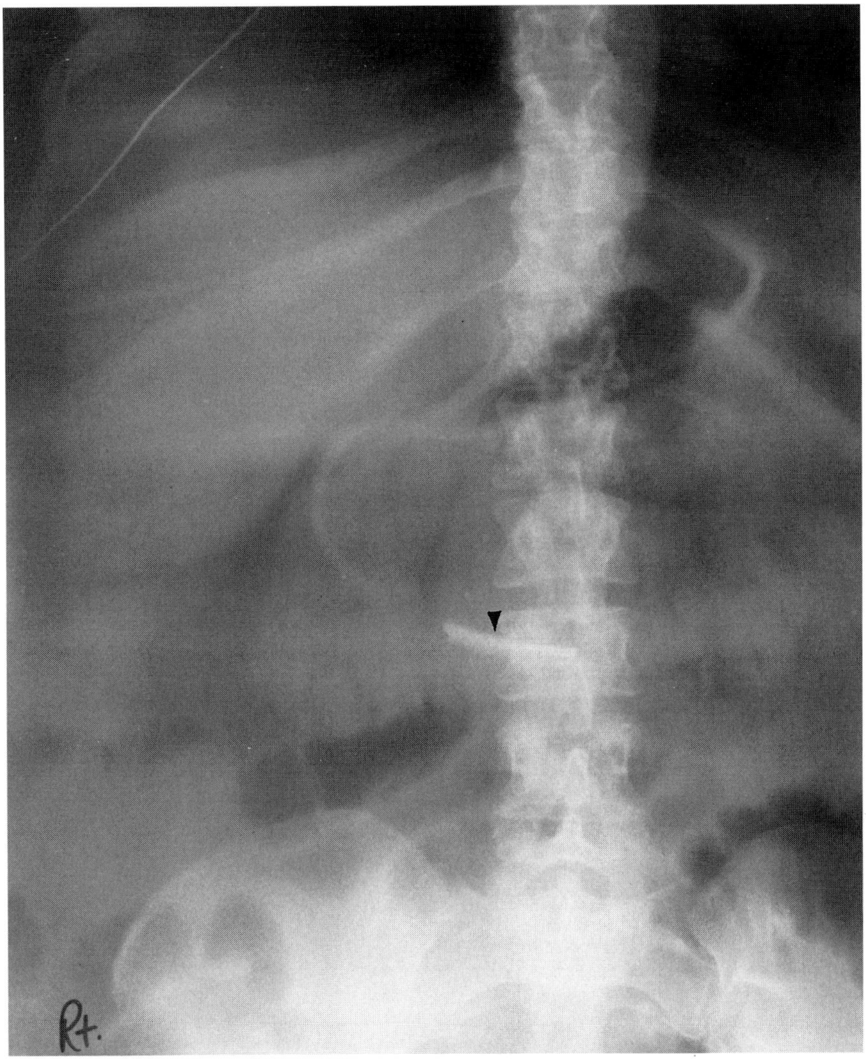

Fig. 5-4 A small bore feeding tube does not contain the traditional radiopaque line. The metallic tip of the tube is evident, and when feedings are infused through the tube, the fluid density in the tube makes the tube more easily visible. Notice that the tip of the tube has passed through the pyloric sphincter into the small bowel. This tube is positioned in the fourth portion of the duodenum.

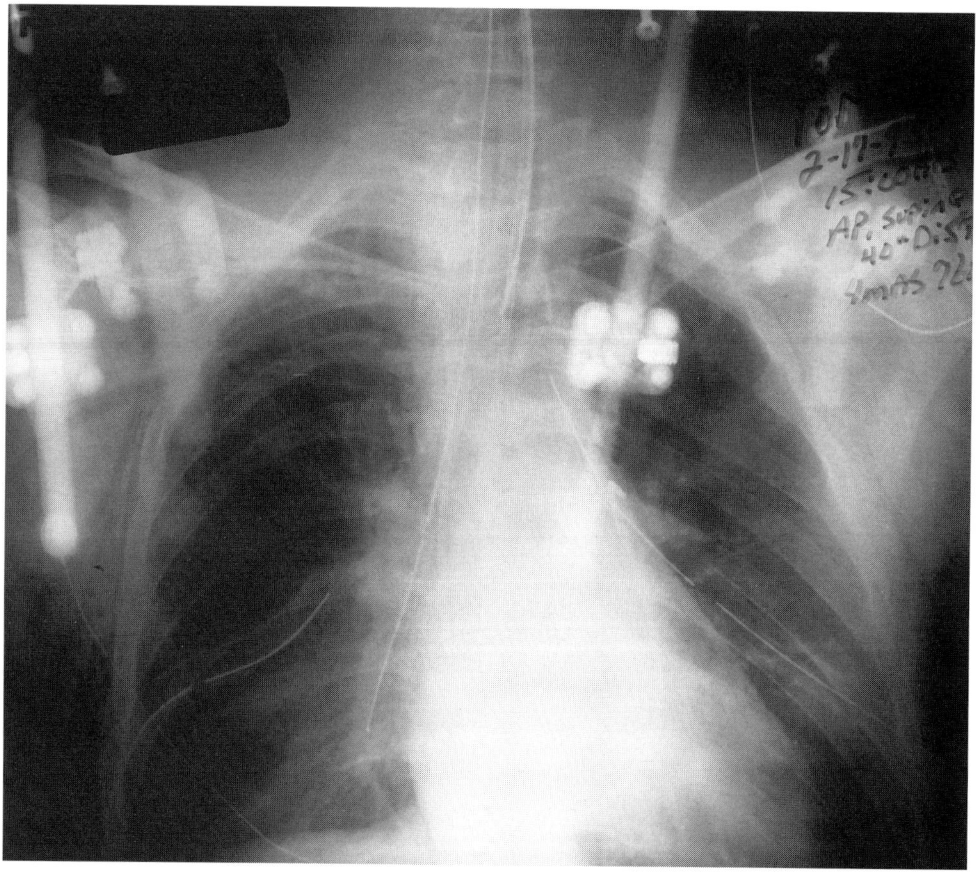

Fig. 5-5 It is easy for the nasogastric or feeding tube to pass into the lung of an intubated patient. Notice how this nasogastric tube follows the endotracheal tube into the lung of this patient. Common sequelae of this incident are a pneumothorax and emergent chest tube insertion.

Nursing Implications

Continuous feedings are generally not instituted in feeding tubes located in the stomach, regardless of the type of tube. The position of the tube should be assessed before the instillation of any fluid or medication. If the nurse observes that the feeding tube is positioned incorrectly, the physician should be notified, especially if the tube is knotted or in the lung.

ILEUS

Definition

An ileus is fairly common in acutely ill patients and it may be mild to severe in intensity. Bowel motility decreases, allowing air, fluids, or food to accumulate in the small intestine. Anesthetics, sedatives, analgesics, infection, sepsis, obstruction, and immobility are among the factors responsible for the development of an ileus.

Clinical Findings

The patient may have an enlarged abdomen. He or she may complain of abdominal pain or fullness, nausea, or vomiting. If the patient is receiving supplemental enteral tube feedings, the nurse should measure elevated gastric residuals; this measurement will indicate if food is not moving through the bowel.

Radiologic Appearance

An ileus is usually observed on an abdominal radiograph, but may also be observed on a chest radiograph. The small bowel appears dilated; the diameter is normally about 2 to 3 cm. If the small bowel is extremely dilated (in most patients a diameter of approximately 10 cm), there is danger of perforation (Fig. 5-6).

Nursing Implications

Patients with an ileus usually require nasogastric decompression and parenteral alimentation. If the ileus is severe, the patient may require the insertion of a double lumen balloon-tipped intestinal tube, such as a Miller-Abbott

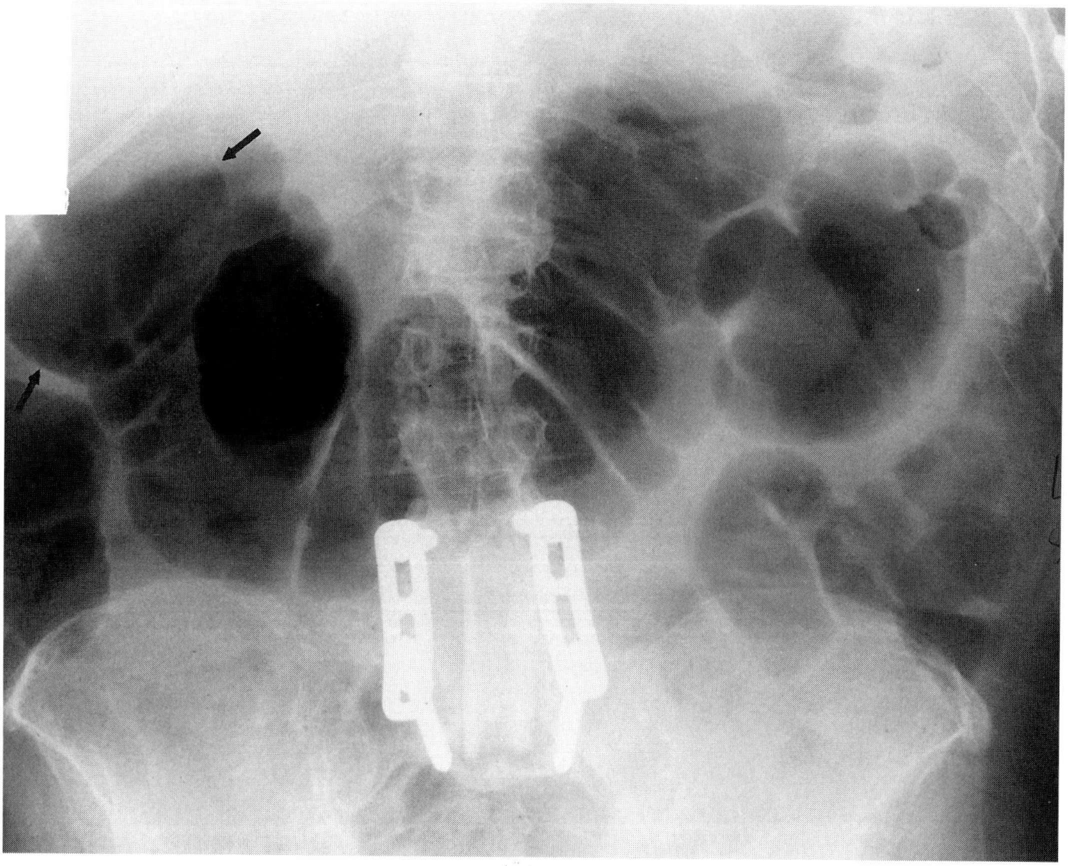

Fig. 5-6 An ileus as viewed with an abdominal radiograph. Notice the dilated loops of bowel. Arrows mark the edge of the bowel. Care must be taken to prevent perforation.

tube. This tube is approximately 6 feet long and contains a mercury-weighted sac.

NASOGASTRIC TUBE

Definition

Nasogastric tubes vary in diameter and have a thin radiopaque line extending the entire length of the tube. Black depth markings appear approximately every 10 cm on the external portion of the tube. In an adult, the most common size used is an 18 Fr. There is a break in the line at the proximal hole, which is approximately 3 inches from the tip of the tube in the adult version. The hole at the tip of the tube usually drains fluid, and the upper hole drains air.

Clinical Findings

The nasogastric tube is inserted to drain fluid and air from the stomach and should be assessed frequently for correct position and functioning. If there is excessive air or fluid in the patient's stomach, the nurse will assess an enlarged gastric region. Percussion will reveal tympany if the stomach is distended with air or dullness if there is excessive fluid. The nurse should assess how much of the nasogastric tube is extending from the nare. In many cases two or three depth markers will be evident between the nare and the proximal end of the tube.

Radiologic Appearance

The nasogastric tube should appear as a straight line that extends from the top of the x-ray film to the stomach, if there is no curvature of the esophagus. The tip of the tube should lie in the lower portion of the stomach near the pylorus (Fig. 5-7). If the nasogastric tube is inserted too far, the nurse will assess one of two tube positions: the tube may pass the pyloric sphincter and extend into the small bowel, or it may loop or curl in the stomach with the tip directed upward toward the fundus resulting in neither hole being in the lower portion of the stomach. Alternately, if the nasogastric tube is not inserted far enough, the tip of the radiopaque line of the nasogastric tube is seen in the esophagus or in the upper portion of the stomach (Fig. 5-8). Occasionally, the surgeon will place a nasogastric tube in a different position under direct vision to avoid sutures or to drain a surgical area. In these cases, the tip of the tube may not be in the positions described here.

In some instances, the nurse may notice that the tip of the nasogastric tube is not in the alimentary tract but in the lung or pleural space. This can occur more often if the patient has an endotracheal tube or is unable to cooperate with insertion. In these cases, the nasogastric tube follows the right or left mainstem bronchus instead of staying in the midline with the esophagus.

Nursing Implications

An incorrectly placed nasogastric tube may result in aspiration of gastric contents, gastric rupture, or instillation of fluids or medications into the thorax. Nothing should be instilled into the nasogastric tube until its position is confirmed by aspiration of gastric contents, confirmation of gastric pH, or examination of the x-ray film. Instillation of an air bolus is no longer considered a verification of correct tube placement. If the tube enters the lung, the result may be a pneumothorax. Excessive coughing during tube insertion may be a clue that the tube is incorrectly positioned, although the tube may enter the lung without clinical signs and symptoms.

PERFORATED BOWEL

Definition

The term *perforated bowel* is often used interchangeably with *perforated viscous* or *ruptured bowel*. It may be the result of an intestinal obstruction, an ulcer that has eroded through the wall of the stomach or small bowel, or blunt, or more commonly, penetrating trauma.

Clinical Findings

Patients with a perforated bowel are very ill. When a perforation occurs, fecal material spills into the peritoneum, causing inflammation and infection. Patients usually have an elevated temperature and other systemic signs of infection, including shock. The patient usually experiences abdominal pain, nausea, vomiting, and abnormal bowel movements. The patient may have a rigid abdomen if there is peritonitis.

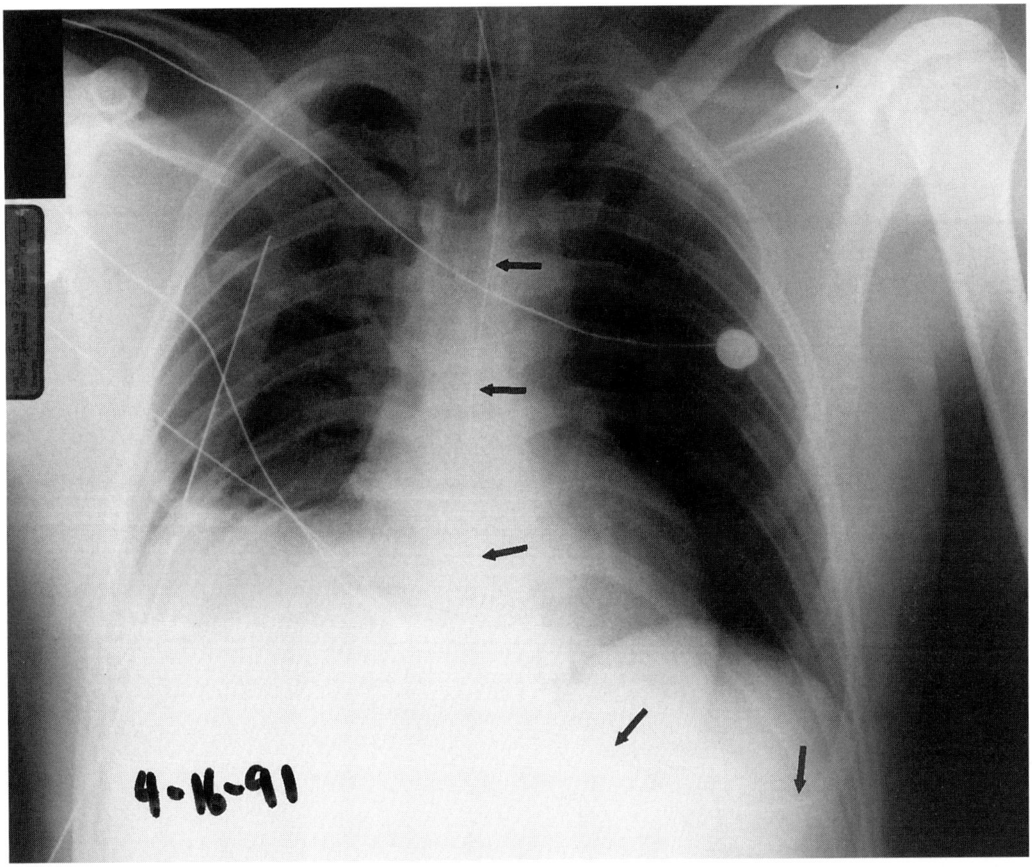

Fig. 5-7 A nasogastric tube is identified by the thin radiopaque line extending the length of the tube; there is a break in the line at the proximal hole. This is an example of a nasogastric tube in good position. Notice that this patient also has a right chest tube and an endotracheal tube.

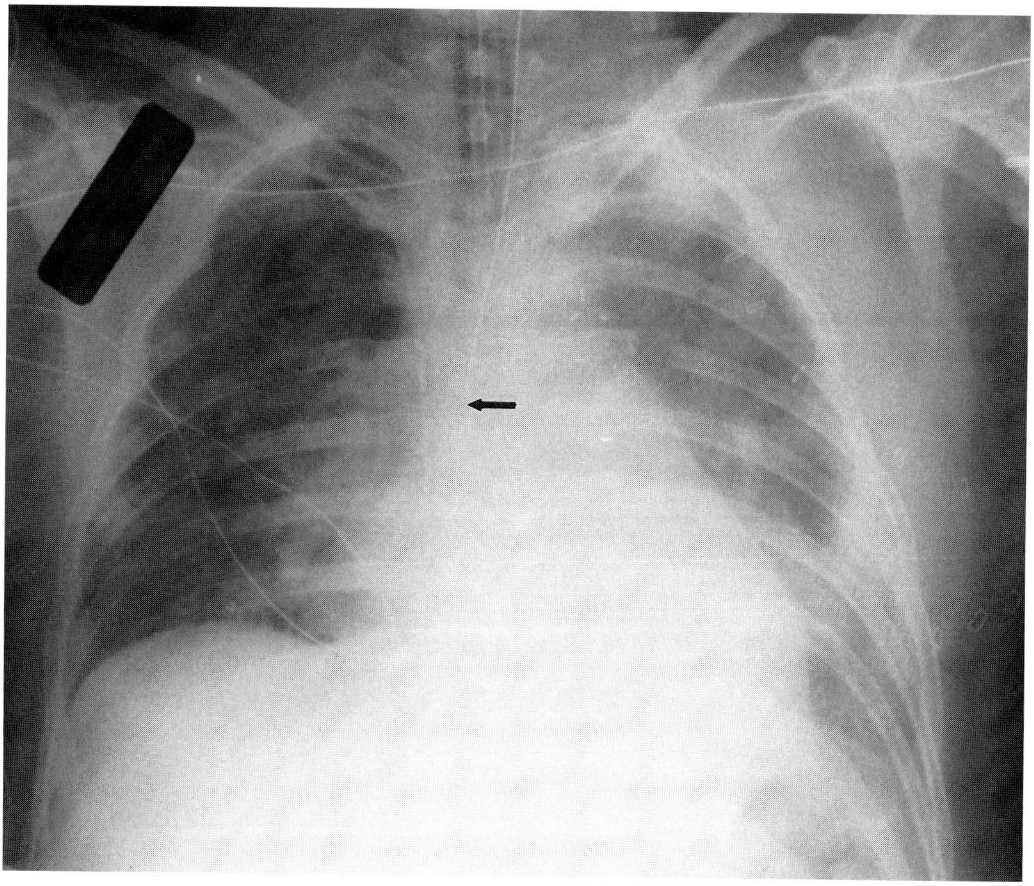

Fig. 5-8 A nasogastric tube in poor position. This patient receives ineffective drainage of stomach contents. Also notice the surgical staples, and that the endotracheal tube is positioned too high.

Radiologic Appearance

The hallmark sign for a bowel perforation is free air under the diaphragm on a chest or abdominal radiograph or free air in the peritoneum on an abdominal radiograph. To obtain the best quality film, the patient should be positioned on the left side (left lateral decubitus) for 10 to 20 minutes to allow air/gas to rise just under the right hemidiaphragm. If the patient is positioned on the right side, the air will rise under the left diaphragm and may be difficult to distinguish from a gastric air bubble (Figs. 5-9 and 5-10).

Nursing Implications

The patient with a perforated bowel requires prompt surgical repair and postoperative antibiotics. If the perforation is not repaired immediately, the patient may develop sepsis and die.

RUPTURED ESOPHAGUS

Definition

A ruptured or torn esophagus is observed following trauma (blunt or penetrating), perforation of an ulcer, or perforation by a blunt instrument such as a nasogastric tube or endoscope. With blunt trauma, acute deceleration tears the esophagus at one of three areas of narrowing: cricoid cartilage, arch of the aorta, or diaphragm. Penetrating trauma, such as a knife or gunshot wound, more commonly causes a torn esophagus. Oral and gastric contents spill into the mediastinum, causing inflammation and infection. The patient may develop mediastinitis, periesophageal abscess, empyema, or peritonitis.

Clinical Findings

A ruptured esophagus is often difficult to detect. The patient has systemic signs of infection, and may experience shock. Acute respiratory distress may be present. The patient often complains of pain that radiates to the shoulder, neck, chest, or abdomen and is resistant to range of motion of the neck. Hoarseness, cough, bleeding from the mouth or nasogastric tube, and difficulty swallowing are possible symptoms.

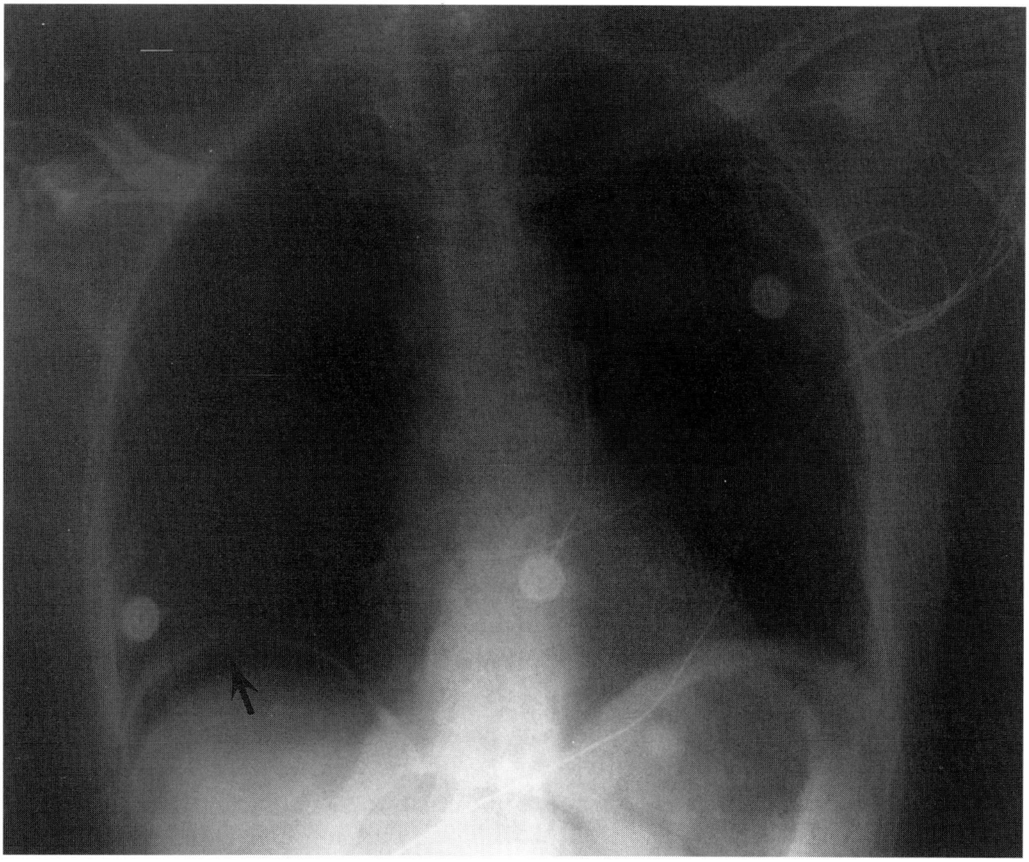

Fig. 5-9 Perforation of the bowel is commonly associated with free air under the diaphragm. Notice the free air collection under the right hemidiaphragm.

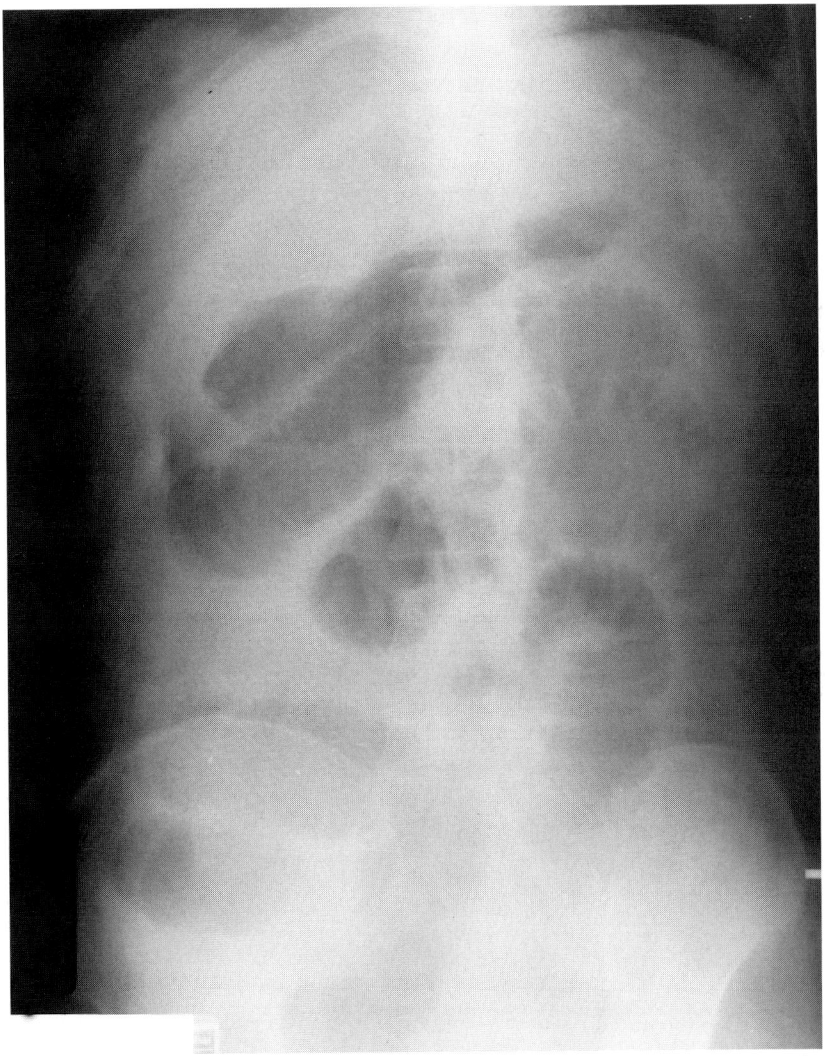

Fig. 5-10 Obstruction looks very different from perforation on a radiograph. Notice the absence of gas in the large bowel in this radiograph. The small bowel is distended. These signs are consistent with small bowel obstruction.

Radiologic Appearance

Often there are no changes on the chest or abdominal radiograph; however, mediastinal or pleural air may be present. The diagnosis is usually made with an endoscope (esophagoscopy). If a barium swallow or esophagram is performed, the perforation extravasates the contrast media (Fig. 5-11).

Nursing Implications

Emergent surgical repair is required. The patient will receive antibiotic therapy postoperatively. Often the surgeon must temporarily close the esophagus and bring the distal portion to the skin surface as a mucous fistula. If this procedure is performed, there will be no nasogastric tube, but the mucous fistula will contain a drainage bag to collect gastric fluids and air. The surgeon usually places an enteral tube for nutritional support for the few months prior to reanastomosis of the esophagus.

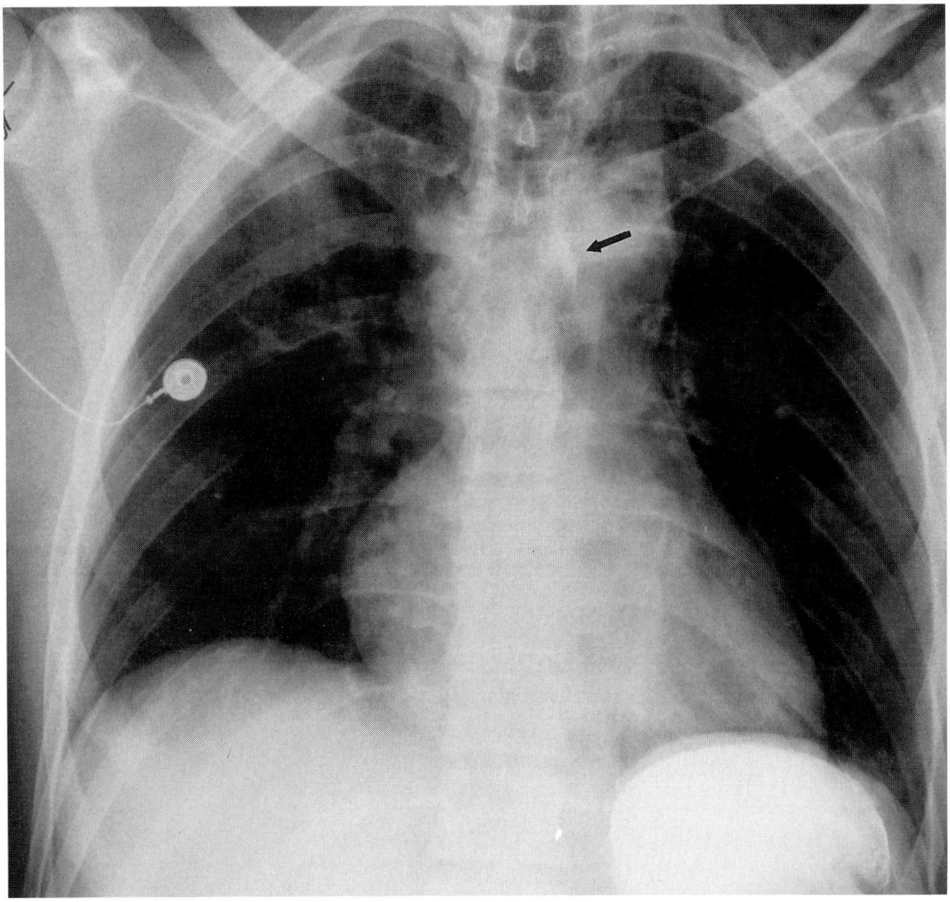

A

Fig. 5-11 **A** through **C,** Esophageal tear. Extravasation of barium just to the left of the trachea can be seen more clearly on **B.** Esophagram window shows the tenting of the loculated leak.

Continued.

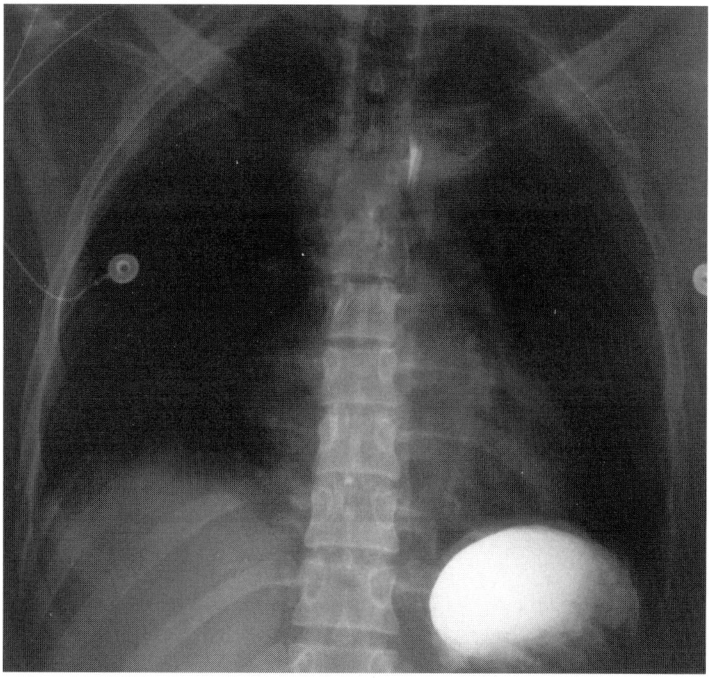

B

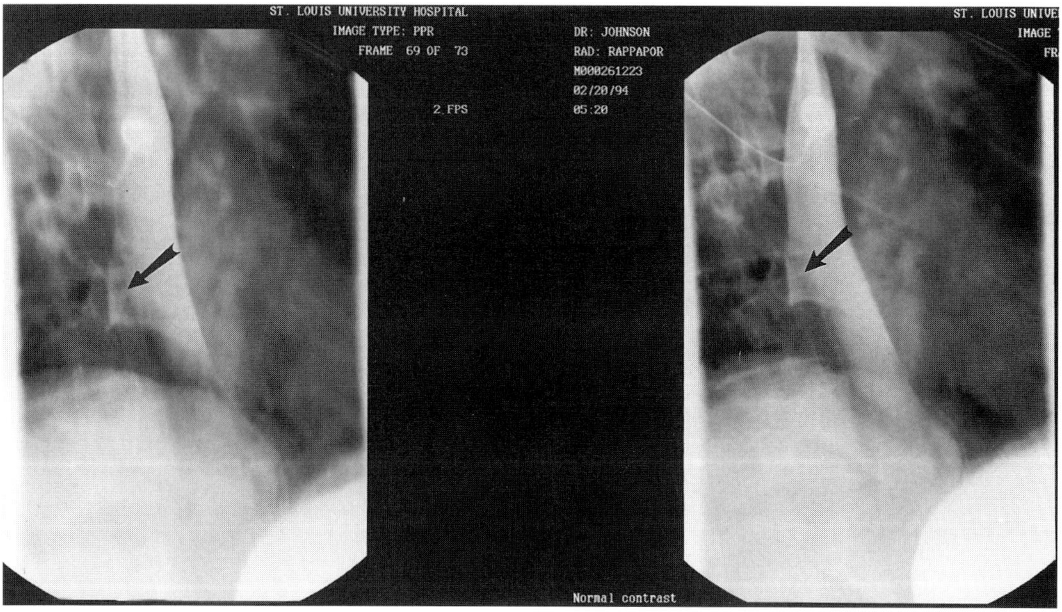

C

Fig. 5-11, cont'd

TEST YOURSELF

Use your knowledge of assessing an abdominal radiograph to answer the questions under Fig. 5-12, A and B.

A

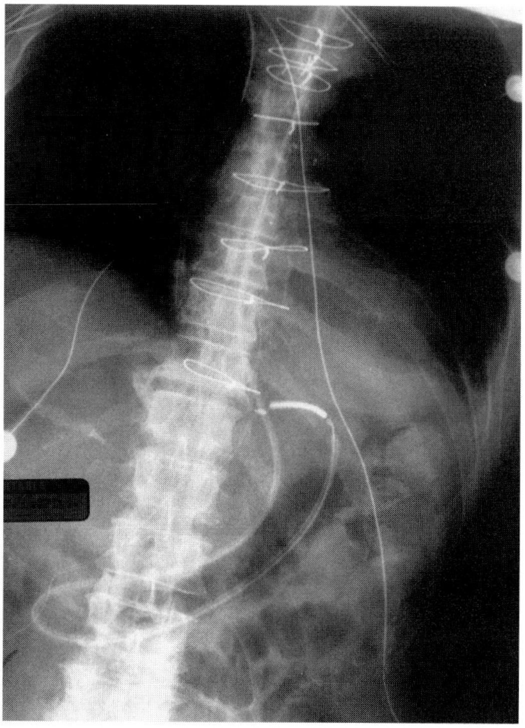

B

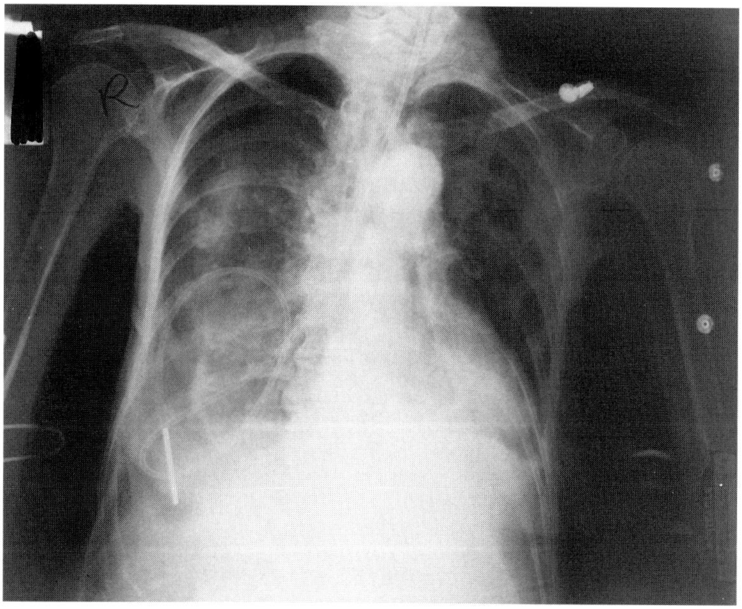

Fig. 5-12 **A,** Is this feeding tube in good position? Should you feed this patient? **B,** Identify the tubing on this radiograph. Should you infuse medicines or alimentation through this tube? What should you do next?

REFERENCE

Ballinger PW: *Merrill's Atlas of radiographic positions and radiologic procedures,* ed 7, St Louis, 1991, Mosby.

APPENDIX

Answers to the Test Yourself sections.

Fig. 3-49. This patient has a knotted pulmonary artery catheter in the right internal jugular vein, which may need to be surgically removed. Also note the infiltrate in the right lower lobe secondary to aspiration.

Fig. 4-27. This patient sustained multiple injuries in a helicopter crash. The CT scan shows multiple facial fractures on the bone windows. Notice the lack of symmetrical structures in the brain windows. The detail demonstrates an extraaxial fluid collection in the left parietal region consistent with a subdural hematoma. There is a mass effect because there is a midline shift of the ventricles. The left ventricles may have herniated under the interhemispheric fissure. Notice the extensive soft-tissue swelling on the right side of the head.

Fig. 5-12. **A,** The feeding tube has coiled in the stomach and is attempting to re-enter the esophagus. This patient should not be fed until the feeding tube is pulled back. **B,** Nothing should be instilled in this feeding tube. It has entered the right lung and is coiled in either the parenchyma or pleural space. There is no evidence of pneumothorax. The feeding tube must be removed. A physician and chest tube insertion set should be available.

Index

A

B

C

F

G

H

I

N

O

P

V

W

X